Seizure and Epilepsy Care

Seizure and Epilepsy Care

The Pocket Epileptologist

Patrick Landazuri
University of Kansas Medical Center

Nuria Lacuey Lecumberri
University of Texas Health Science Center at Houston

Laura Vilella Bertran
University of Texas Health Science Center at Houston

Mark Farrenburg
University of Kansas Medical Center

Samden Lhatoo
University of Texas Health Science Center at Houston

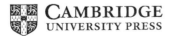

CAMBRIDGE
UNIVERSITY PRESS

CAMBRIDGE
UNIVERSITY PRESS

University Printing House, Cambridge CB2 8BS, United Kingdom

One Liberty Plaza, 20th Floor, New York, NY 10006, USA

477 Williamstown Road, Port Melbourne, VIC 3207, Australia

314–321, 3rd Floor, Plot 3, Splendor Forum, Jasola District Centre,
New Delhi – 110025, India

103 Penang Road, #05–06/07, Visioncrest Commercial, Singapore 238467

Cambridge University Press is part of the University of Cambridge.

It furthers the University's mission by disseminating knowledge in the pursuit of
education, learning, and research at the highest international levels of excellence.

www.cambridge.org
Information on this title: www.cambridge.org/9781009264983
DOI: 10.1017/9781009264976

First published 2023

Printed in the United Kingdom by TJ Books Limited, Padstow Cornwall

A catalogue record for this publication is available from the British Library.

ISBN 978-1-009-26498-3 Paperback

Contents

How Do I Evaluate a First-Time Seizure?

Seeing a patient for a possible first seizure is an everyday consult in both outpatient and inpatient neurology. It is important to recognize that a first seizure is a time of high stress for the patient and their family. Essentially, they will look to you for five "answers" to the following questions:

1. Why did I have a seizure?
2. Will I have more seizures (i.e., do I have epilepsy)?
   a. If I have epilepsy, what kind of epilepsy do I have?
   b. If I do not have epilepsy, what is the diagnosis?
3. What kind of testing do I need to undergo?
4. Do I need to take antiseizure medicines (ASMs), and if so, for how long?
5. How will this affect my life?

To answer these questions, you will first need to answer several other questions for yourself through the history from the patient. To make an accurate diagnosis, the questions you will ask yourself are:

1. What history should I take to make a diagnosis?
2. If it is not a seizure, what are other possible diagnoses?
3. What further work up should I order?
4. Do I need to start an ASM?
5. How do I counsel the patient about their questions?

While ordering objective tests is a routine part of neurological care, *obtaining an excellent history is the most direct and impactful intervention you can make immediately on seeing the patient*. Therefore, this chapter focuses significantly on obtaining a specific epilepsy history that allows you to generate an accurate differential, proceed with an evidence-based evaluation, consider ASM therapy, and provide appropriate counseling to your patient.

Taking the Right History in an Efficient Manner

As with all medical care, obtaining an accurate diagnosis begins with a history. *An accurate history can lead to a specific epilepsy diagnosis nearly 50% of the time,* compared favorably to the diagnosis rate of electroencephalogram (EEG) at 30% [1]. An accurate seizure history can be obtained with essentially two critical pieces of information:

1. A thorough seizure semiology history
2. Assessment of epilepsy or seizure risk factors.

IMPROVING YOUR SEIZURE HISTORY TO EFFICIENTLY UTILIZE YOUR TIME

An accurate seizure semiology history can approximate the brain area that produces clinical symptoms during a patient's seizure, aka the symptomatogenic zone [2]. Seizure semiology is a description of the patient's subjective feelings as well as objective behaviors and movements during seizures. Thus, the first symptom in a patient's seizure description is often, although not always, quite close to where the seizure begins and is of fundamental interest. Therefore, the most important question you can ask a patient is:

What is the first thing that happens when you have a seizure?

When you ask this question, often a patient will begin at the end of the seizure, typically the tonic clonic portion, and likely the most traumatic part of the first seizure experience to patients and their loved ones alike.

It is key to acknowledge the tonic clonic portion as you gently guide the patient back to the beginning of the seizure where often the most localizing history can be obtained.

After establishing the first seizure symptom, it is useful to proceed with questions like: *What happens next?* This question can be asked multiple times until the patient describes the seizure's end.

Once the patient's complete seizure recollection is obtained, one can ask the patient specific questions regarding typical seizure auras (i.e., Do you have strange tastes out of nowhere?) to elicit history of a potential gustatory aura) since many patients do not understand that those symptoms are part of their seizure until identified by you.

Moreover, a history of auras in isolation that precede a first bilateral tonic clonic seizure can establish an epilepsy diagnosis since the patient has already had more than two seizures. Indeed, nearly three-quarters of patients have had "small" seizures prior to a first generalized tonic clonic (GTC) seizure [3]. Identifying this crucial history makes the decision to start ASM therapy straightforward (discussed later in this chapter).

Lastly, clinical history from the period after a seizure concludes (the postictal period) can provide invaluable clues to the patient's epilepsy diagnosis. Here, questions can probe specific neurological dysfunction, the two most common being postictal weakness and aphasia.

Unilateral postictal weakness (Todd's paralysis) reliably lateralizes seizure onset to the brain hemisphere contralateral to the weakness. For example, left postictal weakness lateralizes to the right cerebral hemisphere. Postictal aphasia lateralizes to the language-dominant hemisphere, most commonly the left hemisphere [4].

In summary, a neurologist can divide a seizure into four possible phases as the history is obtained. Doing so can provide further organization that makes understanding a patient's seizure progression more intuitive.

1. A beginning portion where the patient is aware (auras; Table 1.1)
2. A portion where the patient is unaware (Tables 1.2 and 1.3)

Table 1.1 Sensory seizures[a]

Common patient descriptors	Seizure Semiology Classification [5]	2017 seizure classification [6,7]
Déjà vu, panic, anxiety, hallucinations, fear, unease	Psychic aura	Focal aware cognitive seizure *or* Focal aware emotional seizure
Foul smell like rotten eggs, sulfur	Olfactory aura	Focal aware sensory seizure
Sometimes foul or metallic taste	Gustatory aura	Focal aware sensory seizure
Rising or flipping sensation of the stomach, mild nausea	Abdominal aura	Focal aware sensory seizure *or* Focal aware autonomic seizure
Flushing, intense nausea, choking sensation, palpitations, hair standing on end	Autonomic aura	Focal aware autonomic seizure
Tingling, prickling; less commonly numbness	Somatosensory aura	Focal aware sensory seizure
Tones, clicks, basic sounds; less commonly complex sounds like music	Auditory aura	Focal aware sensory seizure
Flashing or swirling lights	Visual aura	Focal aware sensory seizure

Symptoms and the 1998 seizure name should include a laterality modifier when appropriate with options including left, right, axial, or generalized. The 2017 seizure classification does not include laterality modifiers.

[a] Also commonly called auras (focal aware seizures)

Table 1.2 Seizures primarily affecting consciousness/behavior

Common patient descriptors	Seizure Semiology Classification [5]	2017 seizure classification [6, 7]
Unresponsiveness, incorrect answers to questions, space out, blank out, repetitive, or simple responses (yeah, no, etc.)	Dialeptic seizure	Focal behavior arrest seizure *or* Unknown onset behavior arrest seizure
Unresponsiveness, space out, blank out, repetitive, or simple responses (yeah, no, etc.)	Absence seizure	Generalized absence seizure
Lip smacking, "acting weird," repetitive hand/finger movements, drooling, repetitive swallowing	Automotor seizure	Focal automatisms seizure
Flailing, running, kicking, boxing, punching, screaming, "crazy" movements	Hypermotor seizure	Focal hyperkinetic seizure
Laughing, giggling, "creepy" laugh	Gelastic seizure	Focal emotional seizure
Being unable to speak as the primary seizure manifestation with retained awareness	Aphasic seizure	Focal cognitive seizure

All 2017 seizure classification seizures should have either "aware" or "impaired awareness" following focal depending on patient awareness of symptoms.

3. A portion where the seizure propagates throughout the entire brain (secondary generalization with bilateral tonic clonic seizure; Table 1.3)

4. The postictal period (the portion after the seizure concludes).

Table 1.3 Seizures with primary motor manifestations

Common patient descriptors	Seizure Semiology Classification [5]	2017 seizure classification [6, 7]
Stiffen	Tonic	Tonic[a]
Shake	Clonic	Clonic[a]
Head turn, eye turn	Versive	Versive[a]
Muscle jerk	Myoclonic	Myoclonic[a]
Stiffen and shake all over, begin with a loud yell (ictal cry)	Tonic clonic	Tonic clonic
Fall, "just drop," head drop	Atonic	Atonic[a]
Arms stiffen and then hunching over, most commonly in the truncal areas	Epileptic spasm	Generalized onset epileptic spasm *or* Unknown onset epileptic spasm
Can have any variety of previously described seizure types that evolve to a bilateral tonic clonic seizure	n/a[b]	Focal to bilateral tonic clonic seizure

[a] The 2017 seizure classification should be preceded by either focal onset or generalized onset as appropriately determined by other testing except for "tonic clonic" and "epileptic spasm," which can be either generalized or unknown onset while "behavior arrest" can be focal onset or unknown onset.

[b] The 1998 classification does not have a correlate to "focal to bilateral tonic clonic seizure" as the 1998 classification lists all relevant seizure types from which it evolves. Common patient descriptors and 1998 seizure name should include laterality modifiers when appropriate with options including left, right, axial, or generalized. The 2017 seizure classification does not include laterality modifiers.

SEIZURE CLASSIFICATION SYSTEMS

After obtaining the seizure semiology history, you should have a clear narrative of how the patient and bystanders perceived the seizure from beginning to end. You then "translate" the described movements/behaviors of a seizure into specific seizure types from which you can more easily make a localization.

There are two seizure classification systems for seizure semiology that over time have increased in similarity [5, 6]. The Seizure Semiology Classification (SSC) uses semiology on its own without reference to imaging or electrophysiologic data. In essence, the SSC recognizes semiology as its own discrete data point with significant potential to inform a specific epilepsy diagnosis [5].

The International League Against Epilepsy (ILAE) system by contrast combines the seizure type with an electrophysiologic implication (generalized versus focal) as part of the classification itself [6]. Still, removing the electrophysiologic implication from the ILAE seizure classification yields a similar description to the SSC; hence why overlap is increasing.

The SSC additionally benefits from emphasizing the progression of seizure symptoms [8]. For instance, people with temporal lobe epilepsy can have a classic progression of metallic taste (gustatory aura) to unresponsiveness with lip smacking and pill-rolling finger movements (automotor seizure) to a bilateral tonic clonic seizure (aka grand mal seizure, GTC). By contrast, the ILAE system defines each seizure separately without reference to progression, potentially obscuring key information that informs a specific epilepsy diagnosis. The earlier described seizure would be termed a focal to bilateral tonic clonic seizure, unfortunately losing some of the rich description that allows for the localization process so familiar to all neurologists.

Accordingly, a third key difference is that the SSC encourages establishment of a specific anatomic localization whereas the ILAE system, by definition, limits to one of three localizations: focal, generalized, and unknown [6].

All of those factors reviewed, the authors assert that epilepsy patients benefit from a specific and actionable localization or syndrome diagnosis, similar to any neurological diagnosis. Since the SSC urges the neurologist to establish a localization, we will primarily discuss that classification. However, we do appropriately reference the most current ILAE system in Tables 1.1–1.5 recognize that many neurologists use the ILAE system in everyday practice. As noted, it is worth being conversant in both classifications in case patients or other physicians alike use those seizure types. In the end, *what is most important is that the patient receives a specific and actionable diagnosis*, whether epilepsy, nonepileptic events, or a nonneurological diagnosis like syncope.

EVOLUTION OF ILAE SEIZURE TERMINOLOGY

Before further discussing the SSC, it is worth reviewing the evolution of the ILAE seizure classification since previous terminology continues in widespread use. Perhaps the best-known ILAE classification remains the 1981 version [9], which introduced the terms "simple partial" and "complex partial." The 2017 version changes verbiage without substantive change in meaning (Table 1.4). Thus, it is worth being fluent in the 1981 and 2017 ILAE systems since both are used.

Table 1.4 1981 and 2017 ILAE terminology

1981 terms [9]	2017 terms [6]
Partial	Focal
Simple	Aware
Complex	Impaired awareness or unaware
Secondary generalization	Focal to bilateral tonic clonic

SEIZURE SEMIOLOGY CLASSIFICATION SYSTEM

The SSC utilizes common localization elements from other neurological diagnoses like stroke while expanding on localizations specific to epilepsy [5]. It is useful to break down seizures into four main categories, with the fourth category being less common than the first three:

1. Sensory – commonly called auras; these are subjective experiences of which only the patient is aware (Table 1.1)
2. Consciousness – changes in patient behavior or responsiveness that can be objectively observed and, at times, variably noted by the patient. One novel term of note, dialeptic, is introduced by the SSC and means altered awareness/consciousness as the only manifestation of the seizure. An intuitive alternate term to use here is dyscognitive (Table 1.2)
3. Motor – specific stereotyped movements that can be observed and, at times, noted by the patient (Table 1.3)
4. Autonomic – a less common seizure type where symptoms affect the autonomic nervous system, whether subjective (considered an aura, i.e., palpitations) or objective (then considered a seizure, i.e., tachycardia).

For each seizure type, one should describe the localization of the behavior/movement as well as the laterality, if applicable. We provide four examples of how you would translate a patient history into a seizure type with its commensurate localization.

1. A patient tells you their right arm tingles at seizure onset. You would note a right arm somatosensory seizure, which concisely localizes to the left parietal lobe (Tables 1.1 and 1.5).
2. A patient describes flashing lights in the left peripheral vision. You "translate" to a left visual aura with a most likely localization to the right occipital lobe (Tables 1.1 and 1.5).
3. You observe a seizure with stereotyped posture of the left arm extended and the right arm raised/flexed. This seizure type is concisely described as a left asymmetric tonic seizure (since the left arm is

Table 1.5 Typical lateralization and localizations of seizure types and postictal symptoms

Common patient descriptors	Seizure Semiology Classification [5]	Localization [4]
Déjà vu, panic, anxiety, hallucinations, fear, unease	Psychic aura	Temporal lobe; can consider parietal or frontal lobe
Foul smell like rotten eggs, sulfur	Olfactory aura	Temporal lobe; can consider orbitofrontal lobe
Sometimes foul or metallic taste	Gustatory aura	Temporal lobe
Rising or flipping sensation of the stomach; mild nausea	Abdominal aura	Temporal lobe
Flushing, intense nausea, choking sensation, palpitations, hair standing on end	Autonomic aura	Insula
Tingling, prickling; less commonly numbness, far less commonly painful	Somatosensory aura	Contralateral parietal lobe; can consider insula, particularly if painful
Tones, clicks, basic sounds; less commonly complex sounds like music	Auditory aura	Temporal lobe
Flashing or swirling lights	Visual aura	Contralateral occipital lobe
Unresponsiveness, incorrect answers to questions, space out, blank out, repetitive, or simple responses (yeah, no, etc.)	Dialeptic seizure	Not particularly localizing; should consider absence epilepsy in a child
Lip smacking, "acting weird," repetitive hand/finger movements, drooling, repetitive swallowing	Automotor seizure	Temporal lobe is most likely, although this seizure type has been seen in all localizations

Table 1.5 (cont.)

Common patient descriptors	Seizure Semiology Classification [5]	Localization [4]
Flailing, running, kicking, boxing, punching, screaming, "crazy" movements	Hypermotor seizure	Frontal lobe, although can be from alternate localizations; if dystonia is present, it will localize contralateral to the dystonia
Laughing, giggling, "creepy" laugh	Gelastic seizure	Hypothalamic hamartoma; frontal lobe if mechanical laugh; temporal lobe if "emotional"
Stiffen	Tonic seizure	Contralateral motor cortex or supplemental motor area
Shake	Clonic seizure	Contralateral motor cortex
Head turn, eye turn	Versive seizure	Frontal lobe (frontal eye fields)
Muscle jerk	Myoclonic seizure	Generalized
Stiffen and shake all over, begin with a loud yell (ictal cry)	Tonic clonic seizure	If primary seizure type, generalized epilepsy Otherwise, does not localize
Fall, "just drop," head drop	Atonic seizure	Generalized
Arms stiffen and then hunching over, most commonly in the truncal areas	Epileptic spasm	Can be generalized or focal

Symptoms and 1998 seizure name should include laterality modifier when appropriate with options including left, right, axial, or generalized.

extended), which often localizes to the right frontal lobe, but at the least lateralizes to the right hemisphere (Tables 1.3 and 1.5).

4. A patient is observed to have bilateral stiffening of their arms and legs followed by rhythmic shaking of the arms and legs. This would be classified as a GTC seizure or bilateral tonic clonic seizure. It would not have localizing or lateralizing value (Tables 1.3 and 1.5).

ADDITIONAL HISTORY VITAL IN THE CONTEXT OF A POTENTIAL FIRST SEIZURE

While the semiology history is the bulk of seizure-specific history, there are multiple risk factors that you should assess. In essence, these risk factors revolve around ascertaining if your patient has had any brain trauma, whether acquired or developmental. Straightforward questions you can ask the patient include [10]:

1. Was there any difficulty with your birth?
2. Did you develop normally as a child?
3. Have you had any brain or spine infections?
4. Have you had a head injury with loss of consciousness (LOC) and, if so, how long were you unconscious?
5. Is there anyone in your family with epilepsy or seizures?

Infections can predispose to seizures and epilepsy. Early seizures can be seen in 22% of viral encephalitis cases and 10% of patients present with seizures later. Likewise, early seizures can be seen in 13% of patients with bacterial meningitis and 2.4% of patients on a more chronic basis [11].

Head injury can be classified as mild, moderate, or severe. These are determined by length of amnesia or LOC. Mild is <30 minutes, moderate is 0.5–24 hours, and severe is >24 hours. Rate of epilepsy after mild head injury was 1.5 and not statistically significant compared to 2.9 and 17 times more likely for moderate and severe, respectively [12]. It is worth remembering that people with nonepileptic events more commonly had mild head injury [13].

There is a hereditary nature to some epilepsy. Generalized epilepsy can be passed from either the mother or father. For focal epilepsy, the risk is limited more specifically to the mother [14]. Still, in general, most people with epilepsy do not inherit it.

Besides risk factors intrinsic to the patient, you should assess external causes of a seizure, otherwise known as a provoked seizure. Some medications (bupropion, tramadol, cefepime, benzodiazepine rapid/acute withdrawal) are well known to cause isolated seizures [15, 16].

Is It Really a Seizure? The Differential Diagnosis of a First-Time Seizure

Patients who present for evaluation of a possible first seizure most typically have alteration of consciousness. Alternate symptoms can include specific transient neurological dysfunctions such as numbness, visual disturbance, weakness, or difficulty speaking. When discussing the differential of a first seizure, it bears recalling typical features of seizures as discussed earlier. This will help to compare and contrast with alternate diagnostic possibilities.

DIFFERENTIAL #1: NONEPILEPTIC EVENTS

Nonepileptic events are covered extensively in Chapter 10 of this manual. In brief, these are paroxysmal episodes with some resemblance to epilepsy, but with some key differences. Patients with nonepileptic events are more likely [10, 17]:

- To have asymmetric movements
- To have a start/stop quality to the events themselves

- To have events that last longer than seizures (often >5 minutes compared to the <2 minutes for seizures)
- To have their eyes closed during the episodes
- Suggestive to the event starting and stopping
- To have awareness during whole body movements.

DIFFERENTIAL #2: SYNCOPE

Syncope is an acute LOC or near LOC. The key difference is that syncope is due to globally decreased cerebral blood flow whereas a seizure is due to abnormal coordinated brain electrical activity [10].

A common confounder is when people have convulsive movements during a seizure. This is by no means uncommon as myoclonic movements are noted in 60% of patients in one well-documented cohort [18]. Nearly all patients had their eyes open with syncope [18] in similarity to epilepsy but in contrast to nonepileptic events.

From a historical perspective, syncope patients expectedly have autonomic symptoms such as pallor, change in heart rhythm, or sweating [18, 19]. As discussed previously, autonomic symptoms can be present in epilepsy, but are less common compared to syncope in general.

DIFFERENTIAL #3: TRANSIENT ISCHEMIC ATTACK

A focal acute loss of cerebral perfusion can cause a transient ischemic attack (TIA). Crucially, the initial symptom is more likely to be a *loss of function* due to hypoactivity of the brain compared to the relative "gain of function" due to electrical hyperactivation of the brain region during a seizure. One well-documented exception is the limb-shaking TIA. This is seen as episodic limb-shaking episodes contralateral to the occluded carotid artery [20]. Prompt consideration of limb-shaking TIAs in the work up of "EEG negative" focal seizures is indicated.

DIFFERENTIAL #4: MIGRAINE WITH AURA OR BASILAR MIGRAINE

Migraine with aura can have a variety of neurological symptoms including most commonly visual aura as well as less commonly numbness, speech difficulty, weakness, and vertigo. Compared to epilepsy, migraine symptoms are more prolonged and there is of course the subsequent headaches in the majority of migraine patients [10].

DIFFERENTIAL #5: METABOLIC DERANGEMENTS

Alteration of consciousness, encephalopathy, and provoked seizures are commonly seen in periods of either hepatic or uremic encephalopathy [15]. Acute hypoglycemia with blood sugars below 20 can cause GTC seizures and is a particularly relevant consideration in patients with diabetes.

Do I Need to Order Labs, EEG, or Imaging?

While the previously mentioned semiology and epilepsy-specific history is the most accessible way to make a specific diagnosis in a first seizure patient, additional testing is indicated.

LAB WORK

Lab work in general is also covered in Chapter 6. In brief here, routine lab work such as complete metabolic profile (CMP) or complete blood count (CBC) should be obtained to assess for any infection or metabolic derangement. Urinalysis with or without urine toxicology may also be obtained as clinically appropriate. Many first-time seizure patients are otherwise healthy so the routine lab work may be more useful if considering ASM initiation [17].

An ammonia level >80 μmol/L drawn ≤60 minutes after the seizure can correctly classify 80% of episodes between a generalized seizure and focal seizure or nonepileptic event [21]. Given the specific timing requirements, ammonia levels would be of limited utility and not recommended unless drawn within 1 hour of the seizure.

Prolactin is a desired biomarker for seizures, but is only useful if there is a baseline prolactin level >6 hours prior to the episode. In that rare scenario, an elevated prolactin level can distinguish between a generalized and focal seizure, but crucially not between a seizure and syncope or a seizure and a nonepileptic event [10]. As these are the two more common clinical questions being assessed as well as the rare presence of a prolactin level >6 hours prior, we do not recommend prolactin measurement.

ELECTROENCEPHALOGRAM

Patients with a first seizure should have EEG performed. Data do support an increased epileptiform yield if done within 24 hours of the first seizure [1]. When strongly suspecting an epilepsy diagnosis, data also indicate that a >1 hour study will increase the likelihood of capturing an epileptiform finding. Moreover, the same study increased capture of events (epileptic or nonepileptic) after 30 minutes of recording [22]. The utilization of EEG in epilepsy care is covered expansively in Chapter 4.

IMAGING

The utility of imaging in a first seizure is twofold: rule out a neurological emergency and potentially identify the cause of the patient's seizure. To rule out a neurological emergency such as stroke or intracranial hemorrhage, computed tomography (CT) of the head is adequate. To identify more subtle causes of epilepsy like focal cortical dysplasia, hippocampal sclerosis, and so on, a 3 tesla (3T) magnetic resonance imaging (MRI) with an epilepsy protocol has shown to be superior [23, 24]. Thus, if considering MRI, it is worth verifying your facility performs 3T with an epilepsy protocol to enhance the diagnosis rate of the MRI study. Imaging in new onset and chronic epilepsy is covered extensively in Chapter 5.

Do I Need to Start an ASM?

The decision to start an ASM can be more accurately stated "Do I think the patient has epilepsy?" If you do not think that the patient has epilepsy, an ASM will have no clinical benefit. For instance, if a patient has had recurrent seizures due to alcohol withdrawal, the best treatment would be to address the alcoholism. Epilepsy is defined as one of the three following conditions [25]:

1. At least two unprovoked seizures >24 hours apart
2. One unprovoked seizure with a >60% chance of seizure recurrence within 10 years
3. A recognized epilepsy syndrome.

For condition #1, it is critical to consider all of the patient's seizure types. For instance, the patient has had multiple episodes of déjà vu over the past months and comes to you after a first tonic clonic seizure; that patient has had more than two seizures. The epilepsy definition does not require multiple tonic clonic seizures.

Condition #2 arose to better manage patients in clinical situations such as a first seizure and neuroimaging demonstrating a brain tumor concordant with semiology history. Logically, one should not withhold ASM treatment for the patient to have a second seizure just to fulfill the criteria for condition #1.

When you have decided that the patient does have epilepsy, you should start an ASM. While the topic of which ASM and what dose to use will be covered extensively in Chapter 3, data indicate that lamotrigine, zonisamide, and carbamazepine are reasonable options for focal epilepsy whereas valproate is the most effective choice for generalized epilepsy [26, 27]. However, valproate's teratogenic risk and side effect profile certainly influences the selection of valproate as initial therapy [28, 29].

In general, patients who are seizure free tend to be so at lower doses, so you do not need to target the highest dose to achieve a seizure-free outcome [30].

How Do I Counsel Patients after a First Seizure?

This brings us back to the initial questions that patients will ask you in consultation of a first seizure.

WHY DID I HAVE A SEIZURE?

Ideally a combination of history, lab work, and imaging can help provide this answer. You first should establish that the patient really did have a seizure and then provide an etiology if it is known at that time. If you do not know an etiology, it is perfectly acceptable to tell the patient that the cause of the seizure is not determined at this point.

WILL I HAVE MORE SEIZURES?

Again, you should be able to clearly tell the patient if they have epilepsy. If you do think that they have epilepsy, you are likely starting a seizure medicine and you can tell them that around 50% of people with epilepsy are seizure free with their first ASM [31]. For patients with a clear first-time seizure, a metaanalysis of five prospective studies has indicated that the risk is 40% for seizure recurrence [32] – coincidentally why most patients with an isolated first seizure are not started on an ASM.

WHAT KIND OF TESTING DO I NEED TO UNDERGO?

You can counsel patients that they should have a thorough history, an EEG (ideally within 24 hours if feasible), and a 3T MRI with an epilepsy protocol.

DO I NEED TO TAKE ASMs, AND IF SO, FOR HOW LONG?

This question is essentially asking: "Will I have more seizures, or do I have epilepsy?" If you think that they have epilepsy, your patient should take ASMs. The length of ASM treatment depends on your certainty that they have epilepsy and the specific diagnosis that you have made. For instance, childhood absence epilepsy is a common diagnosis in children that most commonly resolves, so you could counsel the patient that they will likely be able to come off medications. Alternately, a patient who has had a stroke and a year later has a first seizure consistent with the area of brain injury, you would counsel that it is less likely that they will come off medications due to the static nature of the injury.

HOW WILL THIS AFFECT MY LIFE?

Answering this question requires sensitivity coupled with straightforwardness, no doubt a delicate balance.

The first specific thing that patients often want to know about is driving. Laws regarding driving after a seizure differ between countries and states. Commonly, patients may resume driving after being 6 months seizure free, although this length may be longer or shorter depending on location. You should ascertain your local laws. You can discuss that seizure freedom at 6 months, 12 months, and 18 months are associated with a relapse rate of 44%, 32%, and 17%, respectively [33]. This can help some patients understand the local laws who are understandably frustrated about the revocation of their driving privileges.

A straightforward way to discuss precautions taken at the time of first seizure are to note that they are made to prevent injury. Thus, in addition to driving, patients are not recommended to take a bath or swim alone (risk of drowning), use power tools (risk of bodily injury), or cook with open flames (risk of fire and burns) until they are 6 months seizure free. Scuba diving and sky diving are commonly restricted completely in the event of an epilepsy diagnosis [34].

Life events that can be encouraged include having a family [35]. In the United States, epilepsy is a protected disability by the American with Disabilities Act and workplace accommodations should be made for these patients [36].

Works Cited

1. MA King, MR Newton, GD Jackson et al. Epileptology of the first-seizure presentation: A clinical, electroencephalographic, and magnetic resonance imaging study of 300 consecutive patients. *Lancet*. 1998;352(9133):1007–11.

2. F Rosenow and H Lüders. Presurgical evaluation of epilepsy. *Brain*. 2001;124(Pt. 9):1683–700.

3. WA Hauser, VE Anderson, RB Loewenson, and SM McRoberts. Seizure recurrence after a first unprovoked seizure. *N Engl J Med*. 1982;307(9):522–8.

4. N Foldvary-Schaefer and K Unnwongse. Localizing and lateralizing features of auras and seizures. *Epilepsy Behav*. 2011;20(2):160–6.

5. H Luders, J Acharya, C Baumgartner et al. Semiological seizure classification. *Epilepsia*. 1998;39(9):1006–13.

6. RS Fisher, JH Cross, JA French et al. Operational classification of seizure types by the International League Against Epilepsy: Position paper of the ILAE Commission for Classification and Terminology. *Epilepsia*. 2017;58(4):522–30.

7. RS Fisher, JH Cross, C D'Souza et al. Instruction manual for the ILAE 2017 operational classification of seizure types. *Epilepsia*. 2017;58(4):531–42.

8. H Lüders, N Akamatsu, S Amina et al. Critique of the 2017 epileptic seizure and epilepsy classifications. *Epilepsia*. 2019;60(6):1032–9.

9. Proposal for revised clinical and electroencephalographic classification of epileptic seizures. From the Commission on Classification and Terminology of the International League Against Epilepsy. *Epilepsia*. 1981;22(4):489–501.

10. JR Gavvala and SU Schuele. New-onset seizure in adults and adolescents: A review. *JAMA*. 2016;316(24):2657–68.

11. JF Annegers, WA Hauser, E Beghi, A Nicolosi, and LT Kurland. The risk of unprovoked seizures after encephalitis and meningitis. *Neurology*. 1988;38(9):1407–10.

12. JF Annegers, WA Hauser, SP Coan, and WA Rocca. A population-based study of seizures after traumatic brain injuries. *N Engl J Med*. 1998;338(1):20–4.

13. E Barry, A Krumholz, GK Bergey et al. Nonepileptic posttraumatic seizures. *Epilepsia*. 1998;39(4):427–31.

14. AL Peljto, C Barker-Cummings, VM Vasoli et al. Familial risk of epilepsy: A population-based study. *Brain*. 2014;137(Pt. 3):795–805.

15. P Beleza. Acute symptomatic seizures: A clinically oriented review. *Neurologist*. 2012;18(3):109–19.

16. R Sutter, S Rüegg, and S Tschudin-Sutter. Seizures as adverse events of antibiotic drugs: A systematic review. *Neurology*. 2015;85(15):1332–41.

17. JA French and TA Pedley. Clinical practice: Initial management of epilepsy. *N Engl J Med*. 2008;359(2):166–76.

18. JG van Dijk, RD Thijs, E van Zwet et al. The semiology of tilt-induced reflex syncope in relation to electroencephalographic changes. *Brain*. 2014;137(Pt. 2):576–85.

19. A McKeon, C Vaughan, and N Delanty. Seizure versus syncope. *Lancet Neurol*. 2006;5(2):171–80.

20. T Yanagihara, DG Piepgras, and DW Klass. Repetitive involuntary movement associated with episodic cerebral ischemia. *Ann Neurol*. 1985;18(2):244–50.

21. R Albadareen, G Gronseth, P Landazuri et al. Postictal ammonia as a biomarker for electrographic convulsive seizures: A prospective study. *Epilepsia*. 2016;57(8):1221–7.

22. DB Burkholder, JW Britton, V Rajasekaran et al. Routine vs extended outpatient EEG for the detection of interictal epileptiform discharges. *Neurology*. 2016;86(16):1524–30.

23. S Knake, C Triantafyllou, LL Wald et al. 3T phased array MRI improves the presurgical evaluation in focal epilepsies: A prospective study. *Neurology*. 2005;65(7):1026–31.

24. J von Oertzen, H Urbach, S Jungbluth et al. Standard magnetic resonance imaging is inadequate for patients with refractory focal epilepsy. *J Neurol Neurosurg Psychiatry*. 2002;73(6):643–7.

25. RS Fisher, C Acevedo, A Arzimanoglou et al. ILAE official report: A practical clinical definition of epilepsy. *Epilepsia*. 2014;55(4):475–82.

26. A Marson, G Burnside, R Appleton et al. The SANAD II study of the effectiveness and cost-effectiveness of levetiracetam, zonisamide, or lamotrigine for newly diagnosed focal epilepsy: An open-label, non-inferiority, multicentre, phase 4, randomised controlled trial. *Lancet*. 2021;397(10282):1363–74.

27. A Marson, G Burnside, R Appleton et al. The SANAD II study of the effectiveness and cost-effectiveness of valproate versus levetiracetam for newly diagnosed generalised and unclassifiable epilepsy: An open-label, non-inferiority, multicentre, phase 4, randomised controlled trial. *Lancet*. 2021;397(10282):1375–86.

28. E Perucca and T Tomson. The pharmacological treatment of epilepsy in adults. *Lancet Neurol*. 2011;10(5):446–56.

29. T Tomson, D Battino, E Bonizzoni et al. Comparative risk of major congenital malformations with eight different antiepileptic drugs: A prospective cohort study of the EURAP registry. *Lancet Neurol*. 2018;17(6):530–8.

30. P Kwan and MJ Brodie. Effectiveness of first antiepileptic drug. *Epilepsia*. 2001;42(10):1255–60.

31. Z Chen, MJ Brodie, D Liew, and P Kwan. Treatment outcomes in patients with newly diagnosed epilepsy treated with established and new antiepileptic drugs: A 30-year longitudinal cohort study. *JAMA Neurol*. 2018;75(3):279–86.

32. AT Berg and S Shinnar. The risk of seizure recurrence following a first unprovoked seizure: A quantitative review. *Neurology*. 1991;41(7):965–72.

33. YM Hart, JW Sander, AL Johnson, and SD Shorvon. National General Practice Study of Epilepsy: Recurrence after a first seizure. *Lancet*. 1990;336(8726):1271–4.

34. NB Fountain and AC May. Epilepsy and athletics. *Clin Sports Med*. 2003;22(3):605–16, x–xi.

35. PB Pennell, JA French, CL Harden et al. Fertility and birth outcomes in women with epilepsy seeking pregnancy. *JAMA Neurol*. 2018;75(8):962–9.

36. A Krumholz, JL Hopp, and AM Sanchez. Counseling epilepsy patients on driving and employment. *Neurol Clin*. 2016;34(2):427–42, ix.

2

How Do I Make an Epilepsy Diagnosis?

Definitions

WHAT IS AN EPILEPTIC SEIZURE?

A seizure is a "transient and single occurrence of signs and/or symptoms due to an abnormal excessive or synchronous neuronal activity in the brain" [1]. Epileptic seizures have a broad range of symptoms that depend on the initial location and propagation of the abnormal brain activity.

There are different categories of epileptic seizures:

- **Provoked seizures**: seizures occurring at the time of a *systemic* insult or in close temporal association with a documented brain insult. In these seizures, there is an identifiable *proximate* cause such as uremia, head injury, anoxia, or stroke, which all immediately precede or are concurrent with the seizure [2]. Provoked seizures are not part of the definition of epilepsy since they are considered to be due to the immediate and cause and do not tend to recur without repetitive provocation. Thus, rather than considering long-term seizure treatment, we immediately address the provoking cause.
- **Unprovoked seizures**: seizures occurring in the absence of a temporary or reversible factor that lowers the threshold and producing a seizure [2].
- **Reflex seizures**: seizures objectively and consistently demonstrated to be provoked by a specific afferent stimulus or by activity of the patient. A specific auditory tone is an example of an elementary stimulus.

Reading epilepsy is a classic, albeit uncommon, example of more elaborate activities that provoke seizures.

HOW IS EPILEPSY DEFINED?

Practical Definition of Epilepsy

Epilepsy is a disease of the brain defined by any of the following conditions [3]:

- At least two unprovoked or reflex seizures that occur >24 hours apart
- One unprovoked or reflex seizure with a probability of further seizures similar to the general recurrence risk after two unprovoked seizures (at least 60%) occurring over the subsequent 10 years. There is no accurate formula to predict risk. However, an abnormal neurological exam, electroencephalogram (EEG), and brain imaging are factors associated with an increased risk of seizure recurrence.
- Diagnosis of an epilepsy syndrome.

Conceptual Definition of Epilepsy

Epilepsy is a disorder of the brain characterized by an enduring predisposition to generate epileptic seizures with specific neurobiological, cognitive, psychological, and social consequences. An epilepsy diagnosis requires the occurrence of at least one epileptic seizure [1].

What Are the Different Types of Epilepsy?

Epilepsy can be broadly separated into two types: generalized and focal. An epilepsy diagnosis is clinically determined with the support of EEG studies. In some instances, brain imaging contributes to the diagnosis.

What Is a Generalized Epilepsy?

Patients with generalized epilepsy have seizure types affecting the whole brain at seizure onset and include tonic clonic, absence, myoclonic, tonic, and atonic seizures [4]. In addition, patients may have typical interictal and/or ictal EEG findings that accompany generalized seizures (i.e., generalized spike and wave complexes).

What Is a Focal Epilepsy?

Patients with focal epilepsy have seizures beginning in just one brain location at onset. Seizure symptoms depend on the brain region involved at seizure onset and propagation [5]. Some focal seizures are only subjective feelings (auras aka focal aware seizures). The EEG may display focal epileptiform and nonepileptiform abnormalities.

How to Make a Diagnosis of Epilepsy?

As discussed in Chapter 1, epilepsy is a clinical diagnosis. Because an epilepsy diagnosis can be stressful and has implications for lifestyle, employment, driving, personal relationships, insurance, and finances, a judicious diagnostic process is essential [6].

Given the importance of a specific diagnosis, we describe a series of cases that illustrate the process of making an accurate epilepsy diagnosis. This process utilizes history, electrophysiology, and imaging data to reinforce diagnostic accuracy.

TAKING AN EPILEPSY HISTORY

An accurate history can be obtained with essentially two critical pieces of information:
1. A thorough seizure semiology description from the patient and witnesses
2. An epilepsy or seizure risk factors assessment.

Seizure semiology (symptoms and signs described by the patient and/ or witnessed that happened at onset, during, and after the seizure) is

essential to distinguish epileptic from nonepileptic seizures. Epileptic
seizures have an abrupt clinical onset and rapid progression of signs and
symptoms; they typically last <2 minutes. Seizure types and classifications
are extensively reviewed in Chapter 1. Eliciting history of underlying risk
factors for epilepsy (e.g., family history, head injuries, brain infections,
febrile seizures, and developmental disorders) is critical in developing a
diagnosis (Table 2.2).

Case #1: Emphasizing Epilepsy History

A 30-year-old right-handed female arrives at the emergency department
with her husband who witnessed an event characterized by abrupt
staring followed by whole body shaking for 2 minutes and urinary
incontinence. After the episode, the patient slept for an hour and woke
up at her baseline. The patient is alert now and recalls having a feeling of
impending doom and a rising sensation from her stomach right before
losing consciousness. She recalled a previous episode in the past and has
a history of two febrile seizures in childhood. The physical examination
shows a lateral tongue laceration. Lab tests, a routine EEG, and magnetic
resonance imaging (MRI) are unremarkable. What is the diagnosis of this
patient?

In this case, the diagnosis of an epileptic seizure is likely based on the
seizure semiology described by the patient. The patient reports a feeling
of impending doom and an epigastric rising sensation are concisely
considered gastric and psychic auras, commonly noted in a temporal lobe
seizure.

In addition, the witness explains the sequence of events with abrupt
loss of awareness ("staring") followed by a probable bilateral tonic clonic
seizure ("whole body shaking"). The presence of urinary incontinence
and lateral tongue biting are other clues to the diagnosis. Patterns of self-
injury (i.e., posterior shoulder dislocations, lateral tongue bite, etc.) can
be sought on physical examination since some patterns are more typically
associated with epileptic seizures [6].

It is crucial to determine if there was any underlying proximate cause of the seizure such as metabolic (hypoglycemia, hyponatremia, high fever, etc.), toxic (e.g., drug intoxication), or head trauma. This would suggest a provoked seizure and NOT epilepsy.

Lab tests are normal and there was no identifiable cause. Therefore, this seizure is classified as an unprovoked seizure. It is also important to determine whether these or similar events have happened in the past, since epilepsy is a diagnosis of repetitive unprovoked seizures.

In this case, although brain MRI and routine EEG were unremarkable, the patient had at least two unprovoked seizures occurring >24 hours apart, confirming the diagnosis of epilepsy. Even more so, her semiology description is strongly suggestive of temporal lobe epilepsy. This can guide further imaging review to specifically examine the temporal lobes on MRI.

THE ROLE OF NEUROIMAGING

All patients after a first seizure need to undergo brain neuroimaging. MRI is the study of choice for detecting causes of epilepsy like mesial temporal sclerosis (MTS), cortical dysplasia, tumor, and infarct. This is extensively discussed in Chapter 5. A CT scan can be performed in emergent situations, when MRI is unavailable or contraindicated, or patients may have claustrophobia.

Case #2: Emphasizing Imaging Findings

A 15-year-old right-handed male comes to the epilepsy clinic with an episode of tingling sensations in his right hand that spread to the rest of the arm and right side of the face within a few seconds. He then felt stiffening of the right arm and his face pulled to the right. Lab tests were normal, a routine EEG reported epileptiform discharges in the left parietal region and brain MRI reported a developmental venous anomaly on the right temporal pole. Is this lesion on the MRI causative of his epilepsy?

A positive MRI needs to be analyzed in the context of the seizure description and EEG findings to avoid inaccurate attribution of epilepsy etiology. The semiology and EEG indicate a seizure focus in the left parietal region given right sensory symptoms and left parietal EEG findings. However, the MRI is discordant with this finding.

In this case, the left parietal epilepsy diagnosis is based on recurrence of unprovoked seizures, semiology description, and epileptiform discharges seen in the EEG. Although there is a right temporal lesion in the MRI, it is unlikely to cause this patient's epilepsy due to discordance with seizure symptoms and epileptiform abnormality location.

THE ROLE OF ELECTROENCEPHALOGRAPHY

Epileptiform abnormalities in the EEG confirms the diagnosis of epilepsy when epilepsy is clinically suspected and helps distinguish between focal or generalized epilepsies. The presence of epileptiform abnormalities after a first seizure is associated with a 2.16-times increased relative risk for seizure recurrence at 1–5 years compared with patients without EEG abnormalities [7]. Thus, epileptiform abnormalities after a first unprovoked seizure are likely diagnostic of epilepsy. On the other hand, a normal EEG does not rule out epilepsy. Use of sleep deprivation, hyperventilation, photic stimulation, and up to four 1-hour EEG studies increases the yield [8, 9].

Case #3: Emphasizing EEG Findings

A 10-year-old male with no past medical history is brought by his father for a first event characterized by sudden stiffening followed by whole body shaking and urinary incontinence. It lasted 3 minutes, followed by confusion and somnolence. The patient denies previous episodes of limb jerking or episodic staring. An EEG is performed that shows 3.5 Hertz generalized spike and wave complexes. Can we make the diagnosis of epilepsy with only one seizure in his lifetime?

This case provides a classic history for a patient with one unprovoked seizure. Due to the presence of epileptiform activity on EEG, a diagnosis of generalized epilepsy may be given.

Epidemiology of Single Seizures and Epilepsy

- One in 26 people will develop epilepsy during their lifetime [10].
- The prevalence of active epilepsy is estimated at 6.38 per 1,000 persons and the annual cumulative incidence is reported to be 67.77 per 100,000 persons.
- The incidence of epilepsy is bimodal, highest in the youngest and oldest age groups.
- In contrast, epilepsy prevalence is lowest in the early ages of life, increasing to its maximum during adolescence and early adulthood, then decreasing after the age of 30, and remaining constant thereafter [11].
- Epilepsy has the second greatest disability-adjusted life years (a measure of disease burden) lost among neurological disorders worldwide [12].
- The prognosis is favorable for most patients with epilepsy and studies have shown that for newly diagnosed epilepsy, between 55 and 68% of patients achieve prolonged seizure remission on antiseizure medicine (ASM) [13].
- Epilepsy is considered resolved for individuals who either had an age-dependent epilepsy syndrome but are now past the applicable age or have remained seizure free for the last 10 years and off ASMs for at least the last 5 years [3].
- The risk of recurrence after a first unprovoked seizure has been examined in numerous observational studies, providing an estimate of 2-year recurrence risk in the range of 40% [14], which increases to 73% after a second unprovoked seizure and 76% after a third seizure [15].

What Is the Natural History of Epilepsy?

WHAT IS THE RISK OF RECURRENCE AFTER A FIRST SEIZURE?

In a landmark prospective population-based cohort study of children and adults, 67% of patients had a recurrence within 12 months of the first seizure and 78% had a recurrence within 36 months [16]. At 12 months, 100% of people with neurological deficit since birth had seizure recurrence. For comparison, seizures within 3 months of an acute brain insult (e.g., head injury or stroke) or in the context or an acute precipitant such as alcohol carried a 40% recurrence risk at 12 months. Age is a significant factor affecting recurrence risk, with the highest risk for patients either under the age of 16 (83% by 36 months) or over the age of 59 (83% by 36 months). Another important factor was the first seizure type, as recurrence risk for focal/partial seizures increased compared to convulsive seizures (94 versus 72% by 36 months) [16].

Recurrence risk after a first seizure further depends on timing. For example, recurrence risk is higher for patients whose when median time between first seizure and first presentation is *within 24 hours* compared to 1 week (Table 2.1). This is likely because patients who have a recurrence

Table 2.1 Risk recurrence by presentation time

Risk recurrence	Presentation time	
	Seen within 24 hours (%)	Seen within 1 week (%)
3 months	32	20
6 months	46	28
12 months	62	39
36 months	71	52

within 1 week are excluded as having multiple seizures, they are no longer considered a first-time seizure.

HOW LIKELY IS REMISSION IN EPILEPSY?

The same prospective landmark study found that 86% of patients with definite epilepsy achieved a remission of 3 years and 68% were seizure-free for 5 years after the diagnosis. For patients with possible/probable epilepsy, the rate increased slightly to 87% for 3 years and 71% for 5 years [17]. In a longitudinal study of epilepsy patients in Rochester, Minnesota, the probability of remission (at least five consecutive years seizure-free) at 20 years after diagnosis was 70% [18].

When patients are not seizure-free, it is important to note most relapses occur soon after a first seizure. Thus, the longer a patient is seizure-free, the less likely they are to relapse. The following data can help counsel patients about relapse risk. While overall relapse rate at 3 years after a first seizure was 78%, relapse rate fell to 44% if there was no relapse after 6 months, 32% after 12 months, and 17% after 18 months [19].

WHAT IS LIFE EXPECTANCY IN EPILEPSY?

Mortality in epilepsy in several studies has been demonstrated to be 2–3 times that of the general population. Patients with generalized tonic clonic seizures (GTCSs) had twice the risk compared to patients without GTCSs [20, 21]. Life expectancy reductions range from 2 years for people with idiopathic/genetic epilepsy to 10 years for people with epileptic encephalopathies. Life expectancy reductions are greatest at initial diagnosis and improve with time [22].

The causes of death in epilepsy patients differ by age.

- Patients under the age of 50 years died more frequently of primary brain tumors, neoplasms other than primary brain tumors, and lung neoplasms.
- Ischemic heart disease, cerebrovascular disease, and pneumonia accounted for most deaths in patients over the age of 50 [21].
- Other causes of death include status epilepticus, sudden unexpected death (SUDEP), burns/trauma sustained during a seizure, and drowning [21].

Sudden Unexpected Death in Epilepsy

WHAT IS SUDEP?

Sudden and unexpected, witnessed or unwitnessed, nontraumatic and nondrowning death in patients with epilepsy, with or without evidence of a seizure and excluding documented status epilepticus, in which postmortem examination does not reveal a toxicologic or anatomic cause for death [23].

HOW COMMON IS SUDEP?

The incidence of SUDEP varies according to the population that is being studied. The incidence in the general epilepsy population is 0.9–2.3 per 1,000 person-years. The group of patients with drug-resistant epilepsy (DRE) have an increased risk, this rises to 1.1–5.9 per 1,000 person-years. The highest incidence of SUDEP is reported in cohorts of epilepsy surgery candidates and those who continue to have GTCSs after surgery [24]. SUDEP causes between 10 and 50% of premature deaths in patients with DRE [24].

RISK FACTORS

The main risk factor for SUDEP is the presence and frequency of GTCSs. Patients with three or more GTCSs per year have 15 times greater odds of SUDEP [25]. Nocturnal seizures (particularly unwitnessed) may also confer risk [26]. Other risk factors include being of the male sex, an early onset of epilepsy, and the duration of epilepsy being >15 years.

COUNSELING PATIENTS ABOUT SUDEP

Patients and families prefer thorough SUDEP counseling, including knowledge of its existence, factors increasing SUDEP risk, and how they can reduce their risk [26]. They also prefer to be educated about SUDEP at the time of diagnosis or shortly after. Face-to-face verbal discussion and supplementary written information is well received and effective in ensuring treatment compliance and interaction [27].

The current most important approach to SUDEP risk-reduction is decreasing seizure frequency, most specifically GTCSs. Specific counseling topics include medical treatment adherence and surgical counseling (including neuromodulation) for drug-resistant patients. Low-certainty evidence suggests nocturnal supervision as an SUDEP risk-mitigation strategy [28]. However, some patients and families may consider it appropriate and feasible.

Two FDA-approved devices, one using electrodermal activity sensing (the Embrace watch) and the other using electromyographic sensing (Brain Sentinel), are used as seizure-detection devices. Evidence that either device reduces SUDEP incidence is not available.

What Are the Risk Factors for Epilepsy?

Table 2.2 Epilepsy risk factors

Perinatal	Postnatal
Small for gestational age	Complex febrile seizures (MTS risk)
Brain developmental defects	Autism spectrum and developmental delay
Inborn errors of metabolism	Stroke
Hypoxic ischemic encephalopathy	Moderate to severe traumatic brain injury
Cerebral palsy	Cerebral infections
	Illicit drug use
	Alzheimer's disease

What Are the Causes of Epilepsy?

The causes of epilepsy can be categorized according to the International League Against Epilepsy classification [4] into:

- Genetic
- Structural
- Metabolic
- Immune
- Infectious
- Unknown: Even after extensive evaluation, up to 60% of epilepsy patients will have an unknown cause.

Some important etiologies are the following.

MESIAL TEMPORAL SCLEROSIS

Seizures for mesial temporal lobe epilepsy (MTLE) classically begin with rising epigastric aura (produced by the seizure spread to the insula), psychic auras (spread to basal temporal region) and olfactory auras (spread to the amygdala). As MTLE seizures progress, loss of awareness occurs, at times with automatisms. After the seizure is over, the patient could have postictal aphasia if the seizure began in the dominant temporal lobe. Epileptiform discharges are seen in the anterior temporal and inferior frontal region in surface EEG [29].

Mesial temporal sclerosis is a highly epileptogenic lesion frequently encountered in the study of patients with drug-resistant MTLE. Seizures arise mainly from the hippocampus. It is pathologically defined as gliosis and loss of neurons in anatomical areas of the mesial temporal lobe: the hippocampus, subiculum, parahippocampal gyrus, and inferomedial temporal cortex [29]. This loss is seen mainly in areas CA1, CA3, and CA4 of the hippocampus with a relative sparing of CA2 and granular cells of the dentate gyrus.

The etiologies of MTS are multiple since the hippocampus can be easily damaged by a variety of noxious stimuli: cerebral trauma, central nervous system infections (encephalitis and meningitis), vascular insults, or toxins [30]. In addition, MTS is linked to the occurrence of febrile status epilepticus [31]. Familial genetic forms are also encountered. Neuropsychological evaluation can show verbal memory changes in dominant temporal lobe epilepsy and visual memory changes with nondominant temporal lobe epilepsy.

FOCAL CORTICAL DYSPLASIA

Focal cortical dysplasias (FCDs) comprise a spectrum of malformations of cortical development. Dysplasias are characterized by disruption of normal cortex cytoarchitecture (e.g., cortical dyslamination) and underlying white matter abnormalities [32]. It can be found in any part of the cortex, have variable size, and may be multifocal.

Focal cortical dysplasias typically present with seizures and less commonly cause other neurological deficit. Seizures often begin in early childhood and are characteristically drug-resistant [33]. A hallmark EEG feature is the presence of focal and rhythmic epileptiform discharges in the scalp EEG, frequently colocalizing with the lesion [33].

Magnetic resonance imaging is important in the clinical assessment of FCD. Radiological signs include:

- Increased cortical thickness, best noted on T1-weighted imaging
- Blurring of the cortical–white matter junction, best noted by increased T2-weighted signal, particularly on FLAIR sequences
- A "transmantle sign" of a radially oriented linear or conical transmantle stripe of T2 hyperintensity, cortical thinning, and localized brain atrophy [33].

TUMORS

Brain tumors account for 5–10% of all epilepsy cases [30]. Low-grade brain tumors (i.e., glioma, desembryoplastic neuroepithelial tumors, ganglioglioma, etc.) are more likely to be epileptogenic compared to high-grade gliomas or metastatic lesions.

TRAUMATIC BRAIN INJURY

Traumatic brain injury (TBI; posttraumatic epilepsy) accounts for 6% of all epilepsy cases [33]. Traumatic brain injury can be classified in many ways. A pragmatic approach is:

- Mild (loss of consciousness/posttraumatic amnesia [PTA] of <30 minutes)
- Moderate (loss of consciousness/PTA of 30 minutes to 24 hours, or skull fracture)
- Severe (loss of consciousness/PTA of >1 day, intracranial bleeding, or parenchymal brain damage).

The standardized incidence ratios of seizures by TBI type are:

- Mild TBI – 1.5 (95% CI 1.0–2.2)

- Moderate TBI – 2.9 (95% CI 1.9–4.1)
- Severe TBI – 17.2 (95% CI 12.3–23.6)

Posttraumatic seizures <1 week after trauma are classified as early (provoked) while seizures >1 week are considered late (unprovoked).

- Late seizures have a higher risk of seizure recurrence and epilepsy development.
- Nearly 40% of late seizures appear within the first 6 months, 50–66% appear within 1 year, and >75% will have appeared within 2 years after injury.
- For severe TBI, the risk of epilepsy remains beyond 10 years after injury [34].

STROKE

Stroke is the most common cause of new onset epilepsy in the elderly, accountable for 30–50% of new onset epilepsy cases [35]. It is important to make the distinction between early poststroke seizures (those that arise from an acute injury and are more likely only acute symptomatic/ provoked) and late poststroke seizures (happening after 7 days and developing from long-lasting cerebral changes and are unprovoked) [36].

As with traumatic epilepsy, the risk of epilepsy increases for late seizures, with a 10-year recurrence risk of 71.5% compared to a 33% risk for patients with early seizures [37]. Stroke increases the risk of epilepsy 17–20 times, with greater risk according to the severity and extent of the infarct, if there has been hemorrhagic transformation, and a cortical location [33].

Works Cited

1. RS Fisher, W van Emde Boas, W Blume et al. Epileptic seizures and epilepsy: Definitions proposed by the International League Against Epilepsy (ILAE) and the International Bureau for Epilepsy (IBE). *Epilepsia.* 2005;46(4):470–2.

2. WA Hauser and E Beghi. First seizure definitions and worldwide incidence and mortality. *Epilepsia*. 2008;49(suppl. 1):8–12.

3. RS Fisher, C Acevedo, A Arzimanoglou et al. ILAE official report: A practical clinical definition of epilepsy. *Epilepsia*. 2014;55(4):475–82.

4. IE Scheffer, S Berkovic, G Capovilla et al. ILAE classification of the epilepsies: Position paper of the ILAE Commission for Classification and Terminology. *Epilepsia*. 2017;58(4):512–21.

5. RS Fisher, JH Cross, JA French et al. Operational classification of seizure types by the International League Against Epilepsy: Position paper of the ILAE Commission for Classification and Terminology. *Epilepsia*. 2017;58(4):522–30.

6. TA Nowacki and JD Jirsch. Evaluation of the first seizure patient: Key points in the history and physical examination. *Seizure*. 2017;49:54–63.

7. A Krumholz, S Shinnar, J French, G Gronseth, and S Wiebe. Evidence-based guideline: Management of an unprovoked first seizure in adults: Report of the Guideline Development Subcommittee of the American Academy of Neurology and the American Epilepsy Society. *Neurology*. 2015;85(17):1526–7.

8. DB Burkholder, JW Britton, V Rajasekaran et al. Routine vs extended outpatient EEG for the detection of interictal epileptiform discharges. *Neurology*. 2016;86(16):1524–30.

9. M Salinsky, R Kanter and RM Dasheiff. Effectiveness of multiple EEGs in supporting the diagnosis of epilepsy: an operational curve. *Epilepsia*. 1987;28(4):331–4.

10. DC Hesdorffer, G Logroscino, EK Benn et al. Estimating risk for developing epilepsy: A population-based study in Rochester, Minnesota. *Neurology*. 2011;76(1):23–7.

11. KM Fiest, KM Sauro, S Wiebe et al. Prevalence and incidence of epilepsy: A systematic review and meta-analysis of international studies. *Neurology*. 2017;88(3):296–303.

12. CJ Murray, T Vos, R Lozano et al. Disability-adjusted life years (DALYs) for 291 diseases and injuries in 21 regions, 1990–2010: A systematic analysis for the Global Burden of Disease Study 2010. *Lancet*. 2012;380(9859):2197–223.

13. G Giussani, V Canelli, E Bianchi et al. Long-term prognosis of epilepsy, prognostic patterns and drug resistance: A population-based study. *Eur J Neurol*. 2016;23(7):1218–27.

14. AT Berg and S Shinnar. The risk of seizure recurrence following a first unprovoked seizure: A quantitative review. *Neurology*. 1991;41(7):965–72.

15. WA Hauser, SS Rich, JR Lee, JF Annegers, and VE Anderson. Risk of recurrent seizures after two unprovoked seizures. *N Engl J Med*. 1998;338(7):429–34.

16. YM Hart, JW Sander, AL Johnson, and SD Shorvon. National General Practice Study of Epilepsy: Recurrence after a first seizure. *Lancet*. 1990;336(8726):1271–4.

17. OC Cockerell, AL Johnson, JW Sander, YM Hart, and SD Shorvon. Remission of epilepsy: Results from the National General Practice Study of Epilepsy. *Lancet*. 1995;346(8968):140–4.

18. JF Annegers, WA Hauser, and LR Elveback. Remission of seizures and relapse in patients with epilepsy. *Epilepsia*. 1979;20(6):729–37.

19. SD Shorvon and DM Goodridge. Longitudinal cohort studies of the prognosis of epilepsy: Contribution of the National General Practice Study of Epilepsy and other studies. *Brain*. 2013;136(pt. 11):3497–510.

20. OC Cockerell, AL Johnson, JW Sander et al. Mortality from epilepsy: Results from a prospective population-based study. *Lancet*. 1994;344(8927):918–21.

21. SD Lhatoo, AL Johnson, DM Goodridge et al. Mortality in epilepsy in the first 11 to 14 years after diagnosis: Multivariate analysis of a long-term, prospective, population-based cohort. *Ann Neurol*. 2001;49(3):336–44.

22. A Gaitatzis, AL Johnson, DW Chadwick, SD Shorvon, and JW Sander. Life expectancy in people with newly diagnosed epilepsy. *Brain*. 2004;127(Pt 11):2427–32.

23. L Nashef. Sudden unexpected death in epilepsy: Terminology and definitions. *Epilepsia*. 1997;38(suppl. 11):S6–S8.

24. S Shorvon and T Tomson. Sudden unexpected death in epilepsy. *Lancet*. 2011;378(9808):2028–38.

25. DC Hesdorffer, T Tomson, E Benn et al. Combined analysis of risk factors for SUDEP. *Epilepsia*. 2011;52(6):1150–9.

26. C Harden, T Tomson, D Gloss et al. Practice guideline summary: Sudden unexpected death in epilepsy Incidence rates and risk factors: Report of the Guideline Development, Dissemination, and Implementation Subcommittee of the American Academy of Neurology and the American Epilepsy Society. *Neurology*. 2017;88(17):1674–80.

27. R Ramachandran Nair and SM Jack. SUDEP: What do adult patients want to know? *Epilepsy Behav*. 2016;64(pt. A):195–9.

28. MJ Maguire, CF Jackson, AG Marson, and SJ Nevitt. Treatments for the prevention of sudden unexpected death in epilepsy (SUDEP). *Cochrane Database Syst Rev*. 2020;4:CD011792.

29. HO Luders. *Textbook of Epilepsy Surgery*. Abingdon: Informa Healthcare; 2008.

30. S Shorvon. *Oxford Textbook of Epilepsy and Epileptic Seizures*. Oxford: Oxford University Pess; 2013.

31. DV Lewis, S Shinnar, DC Hesdorffer et al. Hippocampal sclerosis after febrile status epilepticus: The FEBSTAT study. *Ann Neurol*. 2014;75(2):178–85.

32. PB Crino. Focal cortical dysplasia. *Semin Neurol*. 2015;35(3):201–8.

33. I Blumcke, M Thom, E Aronica et al. The clinicopathologic spectrum of focal cortical dysplasias: A consensus classification proposed by an ad hoc Task Force of the ILAE Diagnostic Methods Commission. *Epilepsia*. 2011;52(1):158–74.

34. JF Annegers, WA Hauser, SP Coan, and WA Rocca. A population-based study of seizures after traumatic brain injuries. *N Engl J Med*. 1998;338(1):20–4.

35. S Liu, W Yu, and Y Lu. The causes of new-onset epilepsy and seizures in the elderly. *Neuropsychiatr Dis Treat*. 2016;12:1425–34.

36. J Zelano, M Holtkamp, N Agarwal et al. How to diagnose and treat post-stroke seizures and epilepsy. *Epileptic Disord*. 2020;22(3):252–63.

37. DC Hesdorffer, EK Benn, GD Cascino, and WA Hauser. Is a first acute symptomatic seizure epilepsy? Mortality and risk for recurrent seizure. *Epilepsia*. 2009;50(5):1102–8.

3

Which Antiseizure Medicines Treat Epilepsy and How Do I Pick?

Introduction

An overview of how antiseizure medicines (ASMs) work begins this chapter. It then moves into a discussion of realistic seizure freedom expectations with ASM therapy when counseling patients. We then review data for ASM efficacy in both focal and generalized epilepsies. These data indicate equivalent ASM efficacies for focal epilepsies while having different tolerabilities. Randomized trials have suggested lamotrigine may have the best balance between efficacy and tolerability [1]. Special note is made of the superiority of divalproex in generalized epilepsies [2, 3]. The chapter then considers ASM selection based on specific patient characteristics, with renal failure on dialysis being an example. Antiseizure medication polytherapy is explored due to its common use in drug-resistant epilepsy (DRE). The chapter then concludes with evidence-based advice on ASM dosing.

ASM Mechanism Overview

An overall comprehension of how ASMs work necessitates recalling that, at its most basic, epilepsy is an electrical disease. As seizures represent spontaneous abnormal excitation and synchronization of neurons [4], ASM treatment should aim to decrease this excitation and synchronization. Antiseizure medicines accordingly either increase inhibitory functions or decrease excitatory mechanisms. This influence is exerted by modulating ion channels or neurotransmitter receptors at the neuronal level. An understanding of how ASMs work *does not require rote and granular memorization* of each ASM mechanism(s). Instead, an understanding of the concepts discussed will better guide your everyday ASM selection and patient care.

ION CHANNELS

Antiseizure medication can cause hyperpolarization (increased negativity) of the neuron. Hyperpolarization leads to decreased neuronal firing, resulting in decreased abnormal excitation and synchronization of neurons. Hyperpolarization is achieved by either affecting outflow of positively charged ions such as sodium (Na^+), potassium (K^+), or calcium (Ca^{2+}) from the neuron or influx of negatively charged ions like chloride (Cl^-) [5].

NEUROTRANSMITTERS

The inhibitory neurotransmitter GABA increases Cl^- channel opening [5]. Glutamate is the primary excitatory neurotransmitter via its NMDA and AMPA receptors [6].

SELECT ASM MECHANISM EXAMPLES

Antiseizure medication targets that increase inhibitory neuronal mechanisms include Na^+ channel and GABA receptors. Classic ASMs blocking the Na^+ channel include carbamazepine and lamotrigine, among many others. Medications that activate GABA receptors prominently include the benzodiazepine and barbiturate classes, although many other medications also at least partially exert influence via GABA.

As levetiracetam is quite commonly used [7], it is worth noting its unique mechanism on the SV2A (synaptic vesicle 2A) receptor. While its mechanism remains unclear, it is thought to have some modulation on Ca^{2+} [8].

Conversely, glutamate is the primary excitatory ion channel. The development of perampanel is the first ASM that specifically blocks glutamate [9, 10].

The understanding of these mechanisms informs a key answer to a typical question from patients: How long do I need to be on ASMs? As ASMs only work by the previously discussed mechanisms while taking the medication, you can easily respond that ASM therapy is required as long as the patient has epilepsy, since, regrettably, ASMs do not have epilepsy-repairing effects.

Table 3.1 is provided as a reference that stratifies ASMs by mechanisms, with some ASMs having multiple mechanisms of action.

Table 3.1 ASMs stratified by mechanism of action

Sodium channel	Blocks	Carbamazepine, eslicarbazepine, felbamate, lacosamide, lamotrigine, oxcarbazepine, phenytoin, rufinamide, topiramate, valproate, zonisamide, cenobamate
Calcium channel	Blocks	Ethosuximide, gabapentin, lamotrigine, oxcarbazepine, pregabalin, phenobarbital, phenytoin, topiramate, valproate, zonisamide
GABA	Increases	Benzodiazepines, phenobarbital, carbamazepine, gabapentin, pregabalin, tiagabine, topiramate, vigabatrin, valproate
Glutamate	Blocks	Perampanel, carbamazepine, felbamate, oxcarbazepine, phenobarbital, topiramate
Carbonic anhydrase	Blocks	Topiramate, zonisamide
SV2A	Blocks	Levetiracetam, brivaracetam
CBD receptor	Blocks	Epiolex[a]

[a] Epidiolex brand name used to differentiate from supplement cannabidiol products

This can be useful when considering ASM polytherapy, which is discussed later in this chapter.

Realistic Expectations of ASM Efficacy

Patients will want to know how likely they are to be seizure-free when taking their ASMs, or more straight forwardly, how successful ASM treatment is. Around 65% of patients are seizure-free after treatment with appropriately selected and dosed ASMs. This is well understood and perhaps best illustrated with data from a Glasgow cohort, extensively reported on by Kwan and Brodie. This cohort demonstrated that 47% of patients are seizure-free with the first ASM, 13% with the second ASM, and 3.7% with the third ASM. *Less than 1% of the cohort was seizure-free after a third ASM* [11, 12]. Long-term follow-up of this cohort has provided durability of the initial reporting, with minimal improvement in seizure-freedom rate after the third ASM, up to 2.1% of patients [7, 13].

These data have led to an *evidenced-based definition of drug-resistant epilepsy as the failure of two appropriately selected and dosed ASMs* [14]. Thus, when counseling patients about using ASMs, whether in new onset epilepsy or in more chronic cases, it is important that patients be counseled about how likely they are to be seizure-free when considering a new ASM. For patients who have failed two or three ASMs, a patient understanding that subsequent medication trials are less likely to result in seizure freedom may well lead them to inquire as to other treatments, such as surgical therapy, which is reviewed in Chapter 8.

Lastly, patients often wonder if newer ASMs have been found more effective compared to older ASMs. This question was recently answered in the 30-year follow-up study of the Kwan and Brodie cohort. In short, there has been no change in seizure-free rates despite varied use of over 12 different ASMs (Table 3.2). Data from head-to-head randomized

Table 3.2 Seizure-free rates stratified by time periods [7]			
	1982–1991	1992–2001	2002–2012
Seizure-free (n)	63% (89)	64% (437)	61% (591)
Continued seizures (n)	37% (53)	36% (247)	39% (378)

controlled trials (RCTs) between ASMs, which will be reviewed later in this chapter, further support a lack of efficacy improvement in newer ASMs compared to older ASMs [15–18].

Choosing an ASM with Your Patient

The decision to start an ASM is a decision that begins with an accurate epilepsy diagnosis that you have already made. Therefore, the real decision making for ASMs is which one to pick and at what dose should therapy start. Selecting an appropriate ASM by patient depends on the following factors:

1. Seizure-control efficacy
2. Side effect profile
3. Patient-specific characteristics (i.e., comorbid renal disease)
4. Cost to the patient.

CHOOSING AN ASM FOR YOUR PATIENT BY EFFICACY

As discussed previously, evidence indicates the efficacy of ASMs has remained unfortunately unchanged over a 30-year period despite extensive drug development and shifting prescribing patterns [7].

As further evidence, four different double blind RCTs in new onset focal epilepsy compared carbamazepine to levetiracetam, zonisamide, eslicarbazepine, and lacosamide, respectively, without finding any different in efficacy [16, 17, 19, 20].

Two separate unblinded RCTs compared standard and new antiepileptic drugs for new onset focal epilepsy (SANAD 1 and SANAD 2). SANAD 1 compared carbamazepine, gabapentin, lamotrigine, oxcarbazepine, and topiramate. From a seizure control standpoint, carbamazepine and lamotrigine were considered most effective while gabapentin was least effective. Oxcarbazepine and topiramate were minimally less effective compared to carbamazepine and lamotrigine [15].

SANAD 2 compared lamotrigine (based on SANAD 1 results), levetiracetam, and zonisamide. This study found lamotrigine and zonisamide equivalent for efficacy at length of time to two-year seizure remission, with lamotrigine superior to levetiracetam. At time to 1-year seizure freedom, lamotrigine was superior to both levetiracetam and zonisamide. The study also examined reasons for ASM failure. Adverse reactions, but not inadequate seizure control, drove likelihood of treatment failure when comparing lamotrigine to both levetiracetam and zonisamide [1].

In summary, randomized data for focal epilepsy suggest no seizure control difference between carbamazepine, lamotrigine, levetiracetam, zonisamide, eslicarbazepine, and lacosamide, again in line with long-term population data [7].

SPECIAL CONSIDERATIONS FOR GENERALIZED EPILEPSY

While no one ASM has been shown to be superior in focal epilepsy, generalized epilepsy does have two specific ASMs (divalproex and ethosuximide) worth reviewing due to their superiority.

Divalproex has been shown in two separate unblinded RCTs examining generalized and unclassified epilepsies to be superior to levetiracetam, lamotrigine, and topiramate, although the topiramate finding was not statistically significant [2, 3].

For absence epilepsy, ethosuximide was found to be superior to lamotrigine and equivalent to divalproex in terms of seizure control [21]. It is important to note that ethosuximide has efficacy for absence seizures due to generalized epilepsy only.

CHOOSING AN ASM FOR YOUR PATIENT BY SIDE EFFECT PROFILE, COST, AND ADMINISTRATION EASE

Since seizure-control efficacy often does not differ significantly between ASMs, more commonly the most relevant aspects of ASM choice revolve around side effects, cost, and ease of use to patient and physician alike. In fact, side effects and ease of use to patient and physicians were two main drivers of continued ASM development [22]. Table 3.3 stratifies ASMs by generation, which can be useful for generalizations made in the following sections. For instance, in general, first- and second-generation

Table 3.3 ASMs stratified by generation	
First generation	Benzodiazepines, **carbamazepine**, phenobarbital, phenytoin, **valproate**[a]
Second generation	Ethosuximide, felbamate, gabapentin, **lamotrigine**, **levetiracetam**, **oxcarbazepine**, pregabalin, rufinamide, tiagabine, topiramate, vigabatrin, **zonisamide**
Third generation	Brivaracetam, cenobamate, Epidiolex,[b] eslicarbazepine, lacosamide, perampanel

Bolded: ASMs often considered in new onset epilepsy
[a] Valproate considered more prominently with generalized epilepsies
[b] Epidiolex brand name used to differentiate from supplement cannabidiol products

ASMs are less expensive and thus more cost effective to patients and health care systems [1].

ASM ADVERSE EVENT CONSIDERATIONS

It is important to appropriately account for tolerability of ASMs since patients will not take medications on which they feel poorly. Noncompliance with ASMs can lead to uncontrolled epilepsy and remains a common cause of breakthrough seizures [23].

A longitudinal cohort found that 15% of ASM prescriptions (504/3,241) were discontinued due to intolerable adverse events (AEs), so decreased patient ASM tolerability is by no means rare. Nervous system symptoms like ataxia, diplopia, and so on (178/504 – 35.3%) account for the highest percentage of AEs. The next four most common AE classes were psychiatric (117/504 – 23.2%), general complaints like fatigue (116/504 – 23%), skin reactions (107/504 – 21.2%), and gastrointestinal complaints (82/504 – 16.3%) [24]. Table 3.4 lists common AEs in select ASMs.

Like efficacy, there has been no change in overall AE incidence over the 30-year follow-up period. However, the incidence of specific AE subtypes has changed. For instance, nervous system AEs have decreased in incidence over the 30-year follow-up while psychiatric AEs (as commonly seen with levetiracetam) have increased during the same

Table 3.4 Common systems affected by select ASMs

Levetiracetam	Psychiatric, general (fatigue)
Lamotrigine	Gastrointestinal, nervous system, skin (Stevens Johnson)
Zonisamide	Psychiatric, gastrointestinal
Oxcarbazepine	Nervous system, gastrointestinal, metabolic (hyponatremia)
Topiramate	Gastrointestinal (weight loss), nervous system, psychiatric
Carbamazepine	Skin, nervous system, bone
Phenytoin	Nervous system, bone
Divalproex	Nervous system, general (weight gain, acne), bone

time period. This suggests that second-generation ASMs are not any better tolerated than first-generation ASMs, but simply have a different AE profile [24].

Lastly, the same longitudinal cohort indicated the likelihood of AEs increases with each subsequent ASM trial after having an ASM-related AE. Women were also noted to have a higher rate of AE compared with men. Lastly, AEs are more likely in older patients, with children have lower AE rates compared with adults and the elderly alike [24]. Similar outcomes were found in a pooled case control study, except for disagreement about age contribution to AE likelihood, as that study found younger patients were more likely to have AEs [25].

When reviewing specific ASM AE rates in RCTs, a similar story emerges to the population data. In general, there is similar overall tolerability between ASMs, with several notable exceptions. In comparison with six other ASMs, lamotrigine is consistently better tolerated [1, 15], with a metaanalysis also indicating improved lamotrigine tolerance in the elderly [26]. One RCT in an elderly population indicated improved levetiracetam tolerance compared to lamotrigine and carbamazepine [27].

ASM EASE OF USE: PHARMACOKINETICS AND DRUG–DRUG INTERACTIONS

The use of ASMs is classically thought of as challenging, which in large part is due to the challenging pharmacokinetics of first-generation ASMs. Those medications included difficulty with dose adjustments due to zero-order kinetics (phenytoin) and autoinduction of metabolism (carbamazepine) as prominent examples. Moreover, first-generation ASMs are metabolized by enzymes that were susceptible to being potentiated or inhibited by the ASM, thus resulting in difficult to manage drug–drug interactions [22].

Second-generation ASMs are easier to use due to improved pharmacokinetics, which has resulted in more streamlined management for patients and physicians alike. Still, while interaction with enzyme-inducing ASMs is less prominent, it remains present in levetiracetam, eslicarbazepine, lacosamide, levetiracetam, perampanel, and topiramate [22].

Lamotrigine is specifically discussed due to its high level of tolerability and ease of use. There are four prominent clinical scenarios where lamotrigine dose adjustments are required.

1. Coadministration with divalproex – Divalproex inhibits lamotrigine metabolism so one must halve the dose of lamotrigine for appropriate patient tolerability as well as vigilance for Stevens Johnson syndrome [22].
2. Increased metabolism with other ASMs – Polytherapy with carbamazepine, phenytoin, and barbiturates all can require increased lamotrigine doses to maintain seizure-control efficacy.
3. Pregnancy – Pregnancy induces faster metabolism of lamotrigine. Monthly levels should be checked with a published algorithm guiding pregnancy management [28].
4. Estrogen – Estrogen-containing medicines (e.g., oral contraceptive pills [OCPs]) can lower lamotrigine blood levels. Conversely, lamotrigine can also decrease OCP effectiveness so increased OCP dosing and/or alternate birth control methods can be considered for women taking lamotrigine.

Lastly, the idea of routine drug levels is examined. A recent RCT compared clinical management with routine ASM levels versus management based on clinical symptoms (i.e., AE or breakthrough seizure) when using lamotrigine, levetiracetam, oxcarbazepine, topiramate, brivaracetam, zonisamide, or pregabalin. This RCT found no difference in AEs or breakthrough seizures in either group, leading the authors to conclude routine ASM level assessment is not of clinical utility, although they noted utility in situations such as pregnancy or ASM noncompliance [29].

ACCOUNTING FOR PATIENT-SPECIFIC FACTORS WHEN SELECTING AN ASM

Most commonly, patients do not have limitations on what can be prescribed based on medical history or concurrently prescribed medications. For these patients, you are essentially picking the ASM based on the aforementioned side effect profile and cost, since seizure-control efficacy again does not significantly vary between ASMs. The most common patient-specific factor that impacts ASM selection is women of childbearing age, which is comprehensively discussed in Chapter 8.

Some patients are limited by systemic disease, most commonly liver or renal disease. For these patients, ASM dosing must be either adjusted or a different ASM selected completely. As noted in Table 3.5, patients with renal failure have far more ASM selection compared to those with liver failure. For patients with renal failure, levetiracetam remains a reasonable choice since levetiracetam is only renally excreted. Thus, dosing can be adjusted or levetiracetam may be given following dialysis since levetiracetam will not be removed until the patient's next dialysis session.

Table 3.5 ASMs stratified by metabolism/excretion	
Hepatic	Benzodiazepines, carbamazepine, cenobamate, Epidiolex,[a] eslicarbazepine, ethosuximide, felbamate, lacosamide, lamotrigine, oxcarbazepine, perampanel, phenobarbital, phenytoin, rufinamide, tiagabine, topiramate, valproate, zonisamide
Renal	Gabapentin, levetiracetam, pregabalin, vigabatrin

[a] Epidiolex brand name used to differentiate from supplement cannabidiol products

ASM Polytherapy

For DRE patients, consideration of using multiple ASMs can be considered. There is little evidence of whether there is improvement in seizure control. Two RCTs examined the use of polytherapy versus monotherapy.

The first trial examined carbamazepine versus carbamazepine plus divalproex in people with new onset epilepsy. There were no differences found in seizure control, systemic side effects, or neurological side effects [30].

The second trial was an RCT that chose ASMs pragmatically. The patient population was patients who failed ASM monotherapy. This allowed physicians to choose the second ASM according to the clinical scenario. Similar to the first trial, this RCT found no difference in seizure control or side effect [31].

Taken together, the decision to proceed with ASM polytherapy should consider the unlikelihood of significantly improved seizure control compared to continued or alternate monotherapy. Still, there are some key pointers to remember when initiating polytherapy.

1. Using two ASMs with the same mechanism (i.e., Na^+ channel medications like oxcarbazepine and lacosamide) is more likely to result in side effect than improved seizure control [32, 33], with a database study showing higher likelihood of emergency room visits/admissions in this polytherapy scenario [34] (refer to Table 3.1 for ASM mechanism listing).

2. In general, using ASMs of different mechanisms is ideal for ASM polytherapy [5].

3. Lamotrigine and divalproex has shown to be a beneficial polytherapy [35], but should be used cautiously due to interaction between the two ASMs.

4. There is no evidence that three ASMs has additional benefit over two ASMs [35].

Choosing the Starting ASM Dose

When selecting the appropriate starting ASM dose, it is key to remember that patients tend to be seizure-free on lower ASM doses. Practically speaking, this means that when you start an ASM, you should aim to start at a subtherapeutic dose and titrate up slowly. With lamotrigine, a common starting dose is 25 mg at night with an increase of 25 mg every 4–7 days (depending on physician preference) with a goal dose of 100 mg or 150 mg twice daily. Supporting this approach is a population study that examined the median dose for seizure-free patients and intolerable side effects (Table 3.6). Note how close seizure-free and intolerable AE doses are, indicating the imperative to use the lowest dose possible.

The efficacy of lower dosing for ASMs has been affirmed in subsequent RCTs in new onset epilepsy populations investigating levetiracetam, zonisamide, and eslicarbazepine [17, 19, 20].

Table 3.6 Comparison of average ASM dose for seizure freedom versus intolerable side effects

	Lamotrigine (mg)	Carbamazepine (mg)	Divalproex (mg)
Seizure-free	187.5	600	1,000
Intolerable AE	300	400	800

Conclusions

Antiseizure medicines are a very effective therapy, with around two out of three patients being seizure-free with appropriately selected and dosed ASMs. Still, it is important to remember that failing two ASMs unfortunately already places the patient in the drug-resistant category.

The most common seizure-free dose tends to be on the lower side. Monotherapy is no worse than polytherapy with regards to seizure control and AEs. Antiseizure-medication selection should be guided by tolerability and ease of use, as for the most part, there is not a substantial difference in seizure-control efficacy. The clear exception is divalproex with improved seizure-control efficacy in generalized epilepsy diagnoses.

Works Cited

1. A Marson, G Burnside, R Appleton et al. The SANAD II study of the effectiveness and cost-effectiveness of levetiracetam, zonisamide, or lamotrigine for newly diagnosed focal epilepsy: An open-label, non-inferiority, multicentre, phase 4, randomised controlled trial. *Lancet.* 2021;397(10282):1363–74.

2. AG Marson, AM Al-Kharusi, M Alwaidh et al. The SANAD study of effectiveness of valproate, lamotrigine, or topiramate for generalised and unclassifiable epilepsy: An unblinded randomised controlled trial. *Lancet.* 2007;369(9566):1016–26.

3. A Marson, G Burnside, R Appleton et al. The SANAD II study of the effectiveness and cost-effectiveness of valproate versus levetiracetam for newly diagnosed generalised and unclassifiable epilepsy: An open-label, non-inferiority, multicentre, phase 4, randomised controlled trial. *Lancet.* 2021;397(10282):1375–86.

4. P Jiruska, M de Curtis, JG Jefferys et al. Synchronization and desynchronization in epilepsy: controversies and hypotheses. *J Physiol.* 2013;591(4):787–97.

5. BW Abou-Khalil. Update on antiepileptic drugs 2019. *Continuum.* 2019;25(2):508–36.

6. M Steffens, HJ Huppertz, J Zentner, E Chauzit, and TJ Feuerstein. Unchanged glutamine synthetase activity and increased NMDA receptor density in epileptic human neocortex: Implications for the pathophysiology of epilepsy. *Neurochem Int.* 2005;47(6):379–84.

7. Z Chen, MJ Brodie, D Liew, and P Kwan. Treatment outcomes in patients with newly diagnosed epilepsy treated with established and new antiepileptic drugs: A 30-year longitudinal cohort study. *JAMA Neurol.* 2018;75(3):279–86.

8. K Tokudome, T Okumura, S Shimizu et al. Synaptic vesicle glycoprotein 2A (SV2A) regulates kindling epileptogenesis via GABAergic neurotransmission. *Sci Rep.* 2016;6:27420.

9. GL Krauss, JM Serratosa, V Villanueva et al. Randomized phase III study 306: Adjunctive perampanel for refractory partial-onset seizures. *Neurology.* 2012;78(18):1408–15.

10. JA French, GL Krauss, V Biton et al. Adjunctive perampanel for refractory partial-onset seizures: Randomized phase III study 304. *Neurology*. 2012;79(6):589–96.

11. P Kwan and MJ Brodie. Early identification of refractory epilepsy. *N Engl J Med*. 2000;342(5):314–19.

12. P Kwan and MJ Brodie. Effectiveness of first antiepileptic drug. *Epilepsia*. 2001;42(10):1255–60.

13. MJ Brodie, SJ Barry, GA Bamagous, JD Norrie and P Kwan. Patterns of treatment response in newly diagnosed epilepsy. *Neurology*. 2012;78(20):1548–54.

14. P Kwan, A Arzimanoglou, AT Berg et al. Definition of drug resistant epilepsy: Consensus proposal by the ad hoc Task Force of the ILAE Commission on Therapeutic Strategies. *Epilepsia*. 2010;51(6):1069–77.

15. AG Marson, AM Al-Kharusi, M Alwaidh et al. The SANAD study of effectiveness of carbamazepine, gabapentin, lamotrigine, oxcarbazepine, or topiramate for treatment of partial epilepsy: An unblinded randomised controlled trial. *Lancet*. 2007;369(9566):1000–15.

16. M Baulac, F Rosenow, M Toledo et al. Efficacy, safety, and tolerability of lacosamide monotherapy versus controlled-release carbamazepine in patients with newly diagnosed epilepsy: A phase 3, randomised, double-blind, non-inferiority trial. *Lancet Neurol*. 2017;16(1):43–54.

17. E Trinka, E Ben-Menachem, PA Kowacs et al. Efficacy and safety of eslicarbazepine acetate versus controlled-release carbamazepine monotherapy in newly diagnosed epilepsy: A phase III double-blind, randomized, parallel-group, multicenter study. *Epilepsia*. 2018;59(2):479–91.

18. E Trinka, AG Marson, W van Paesschen et al. KOMET: An unblinded, randomised, two parallel-group, stratified trial comparing the effectiveness of levetiracetam with controlled-release carbamazepine and extended-release sodium valproate as monotherapy in patients with newly diagnosed epilepsy. *J Neurol Neurosurg Psychiatry*. 2013;84(10):1138–47.

19. MJ Brodie, E Perucca, P Ryvlin, E Ben-Menachem, and HJ Meencke. Comparison of levetiracetam and controlled-release carbamazepine in newly diagnosed epilepsy. *Neurology*. 2007;68(6):402–8.

20. M Baulac, MJ Brodie, A Patten, J Segieth, and L Giorgi. Efficacy and tolerability of zonisamide versus controlled-release carbamazepine for newly diagnosed partial epilepsy: A phase 3, randomised, double-blind, non-inferiority trial. *Lancet Neurol*. 2012;11(7):579–88.

21. TA Glauser, A Cnaan, S Shinnar et al. Ethosuximide, valproic acid, and lamotrigine in childhood absence epilepsy: Initial monotherapy outcomes at 12 months. *Epilepsia*. 2013;54(1):141–55.

22. E Perucca, MJ Brodie, P Kwan, and T Tomson. 30 years of second-generation antiseizure medications: Impact and future perspectives. *Lancet Neurol.* 2020;19(6):544–56.

23. R Manjunath, KL Davis, SD Candrilli, and AB Ettinger. Association of antiepileptic drug nonadherence with risk of seizures in adults with epilepsy. *Epilepsy Behav.* 2009;14(2):372–8.

24. BAA Alsfouk, MJ Brodie, M Walters, P Kwan, and Z Chen. Tolerability of antiseizure medications in individuals with newly diagnosed epilepsy. *JAMA Neurol.* 2020;77(5):574–81.

25. E Perucca and T Tomson. The pharmacological treatment of epilepsy in adults. *Lancet Neurol.* 2011;10(5):446–56.

26. N Lezaic, G Gore, CB Josephson et al. The medical treatment of epilepsy in the elderly: A systematic review and meta-analysis. *Epilepsia.* 2019;60(7):1325–40.

27. KJ Werhahn, E Trinka, J Dobesberger et al. A randomized, double-blind comparison of antiepileptic drug treatment in the elderly with new-onset focal epilepsy. *Epilepsia.* 2015;56(3):450–9.

28. A Sabers. Algorithm for lamotrigine dose adjustment before, during, and after pregnancy. *Acta Neurol Scand.* 2012;126(1):e1–e4.

29. I Aícua-Rapún, P André, AO Rossetti et al. Therapeutic drug monitoring of newer antiepileptic drugs: A randomized trial for dosage adjustment. *Ann Neurol.* 2020;87(1):22–9.

30. CL Deckers, YA Hekster, A Keyser et al. Monotherapy versus polytherapy for epilepsy: A multicenter double-blind randomized study. *Epilepsia.* 2001;42(11):1387–94.

31. E Beghi, G Gatti, C Tonini et al. Adjunctive therapy versus alternative monotherapy in patients with partial epilepsy failing on a single drug: A multicentre, randomised, pragmatic controlled trial. *Epilepsy Res.* 2003;57(1):1–13.

32. B Abou-Khalil. Selecting rational drug combinations in epilepsy. *CNS Drugs.* 2017;31(10):835–44.

33. EM Sarhan, MC Walker, and C Selai. Evidence for efficacy of combination of antiepileptic drugs in treatment of epilepsy. *J Neurol. Res.* 2016;5(6):267–76.

34. JM Margolis, BC Chu, ZJ Wang, R Copher, and JE Cavazos. Effectiveness of antiepileptic drug combination therapy for partial-onset seizures based on mechanisms of action. *JAMA Neurol.* 2014;71(8):985–93.

35. NP Poolos, LN Warner, SZ Humphreys, and S Williams. Comparative efficacy of combination drug therapy in refractory epilepsy. *Neurology.* 2012;78(1):62–8.

4

How Can I Best Use EEG for Treating Epilepsy Patients?

What Are the Types of EEG and Which One Should I Order?

ROUTINE ELECTROENCEPHALOGRAM

A routine electroencephalogram (EEG) consists of a 25-minute EEG recording. The indications depend on the clinical scenario.

Outpatient Indications for a Routine EEG

- Determining epilepsy type (i.e., focal versus generalized, specific epilepsy syndrome)
- Prognosticate risk of seizure recurrence (after a first unprovoked seizure or prior to weaning medications)
- For differential diagnosis of paroxysmal events such as differentiating epileptic from nonepileptic events (e.g., syncope, movement disorders, migraine, psychogenic seizures).

Inpatient Indications for a Routine EEG

- Evaluation of patients with unexplained encephalopathy
- Confirming an epilepsy or acute seizure/status epilepticus diagnosis
- Prognostication of coma patients
- To establish electrocerebral inactivity in support of a "brain death" diagnosis in patients with compatible clinical exam and apnea test.

It is important to know that only 29–55% of epilepsy patients have epileptiform abnormalities in a first routine outpatient EEG [1], but the yield increases to 59–82% by repeating up to four routine EEGs [2, 3], or in other words, performing extended EEG.

EXTENDED EEG

An extended EEG involves a 30–60-minute recording. It can be requested in association with sleep deprivation. This requires the patient to sleep less than usual the night before undergoing the test. The aim of sleep deprivation is to capture sleep state during the EEG recording, which potentially increases the yield of epileptiform abnormalities detection to 77% [4].

When to Order an Extended EEG

- For patients with higher suspicion for an epilepsy diagnosis
- To increase the diagnostic yield of patients with a normal routine EEG by increasing the likelihood of identifying interictal epileptiform abnormalities
- To evaluate patients with very frequent paroxysmal events so continuous long-term monitoring may be avoided [1].

CONTINUOUS EEG MONITORING

Continuous EEG monitoring lasts from 60 minutes to days of recording and can be done in the inpatient or outpatient setting.

Inpatient Monitoring

Inpatient long-term monitoring indications depend on the clinical setting.

- Intensive Care Unit (ICU) – for the detection of subclinical/nonconvulsive seizures in patients with encephalopathy:
  - During or following convulsive status epilepticus

- After an acute brain insult (e.g., trauma, hemorrhage, anoxic injury)
- For monitoring patients in a pharmacologically induced coma.
- Epilepsy Monitoring Unit (EMU) – usually carried out with medication tapering or cessation.
  - Diagnostic evaluation in patients with drug-resistant epilepsy (DRE), particularly in the presurgical evaluation period
  - Rapid treatment changes in patients with poorly controlled epilepsy
  - Intracranial EEG evaluation of DRE patients
  - Investigation of suspected nonepileptic events
- Operating Room – during procedures that may intentionally or unintentionally compromise brain tissue such as carotid endarterectomy, intracranial aneurysm intervention, balloon occlusion, or the Wada test.

Outpatient Monitoring

Outpatient/ambulatory long-term monitoring indications are often narrower.

- To increase the yield of epileptiform abnormalities detection in patients with a previous normal routine and/or sleep-deprived EEG, where avoidance of hospitalization is desired
- To evaluate patients with frequent paroxysmal events who do not require antiepileptic medication tapering.

What Is an EEG Montage?

An EEG montage is the system by which EEG electrodes are arranged in a systematic and broadly agreed fashion to enable an efficient and accurate reading of the EEG signal. In the 10–20 system, electrodes are named according to the scalp/brain location underlying the electrode. Left-sided electrodes are designated with odd numbers while right-sided electrodes are even numbers. The larger the number, the further away from the midline is the electrode. Midline electrodes are denoted with a "z" (i.e., Fz, Cz, etc.).

Montages are either bipolar or referential. Bipolar montages signify measuring the difference between potentials of two adjacent electrodes. Localizations are made by identifying a *phase reversal*, simply identified as two waves pointing toward or away from one another on the EEG. Conversely, a referential montage measures potentials between the electrode of interest and a reference common to each electrode. An ideal reference will be electrically neutral. For referential montages, localizations are in the electrode with the waveform of highest amplitude.

What Are Normal EEG Findings?

Different awake (Table 4.1) and sleep (Table 4.2) patterns and a number of physiological variants can be seen in a normal EEG. Some of normal findings can be mistaken for abnormal activity and may lead to overinterpretation of the EEG.

Table 4.1 Typical frequencies in EEG

	Frequency (Hz)	Features
Beta	>13 and <40	Seen more prominently in anterior sites. It emerges with eye opening or mental exertion.
Alpha	8–13	Alpha frequencies can be found in any brain region. However, the most common alpha range frequency location is posteriorly. When there, it is termed "posterior dominant rhythm" (PDR) and emerges when the eyes are closed with relaxation (Fig. 4.1).
Mu	7–12	Comb-shaped rhythm. Right or left central region (maximum at electrodes C3 or C4). It is attenuated by thoughts or movements (Fig. 4.2).
Theta	>4 to <8	More pronounced in drowsiness. Normal intermittent temporal over 40 years of age.
Delta	0.5 to ≤4	Slow waves seen diffusely during stage III and IV of sleep.

Table 4.2 Normal sleep structures

Findings	Sleep stage	Features
Vertex waves	I–II	Biphasic, sharp transients with negativity polarity. More prominent in central leads [5, 6].
Positive occipital sharp transient of sleep (POSTS)	I–III	More prominent in occipital leads with positive polarity. Seen in younger adults. Asymmetries are found in over a third of subjects. May occur in isolation or in runs (Fig. 4.3) [7].
Sleep spindles	II–III	Bursts of 12–14 Hz activity lasting 0.5–1.5 seconds (Fig. 4.3) [8].
K complex	II	Biphasic waves with an initial negative followed by a slow positive component, often ending in sleep spindles. Duration of ≥0.5 seconds (Fig. 4.3) [8].

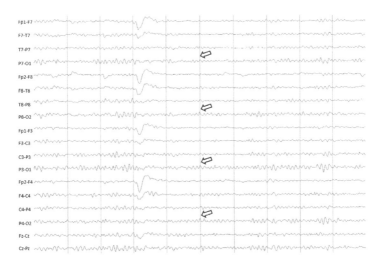

Fig. 4.1 Posterior dominant rhythm (PDR). Alpha rhythm prominent in posterior sites. It emerges with closing of the eyes and with relaxation.

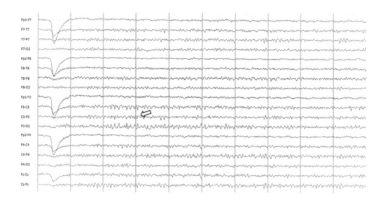

Fig. 4.2 Mu rhythm. Comb shape. Left central region (maximum at C3). It is attenuated by contralateral movement or even thoughts of contralateral movements.

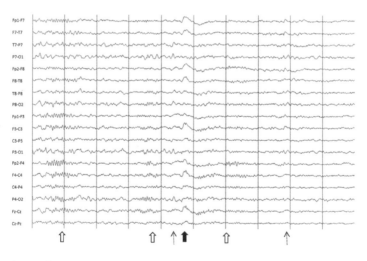

Fig. 4.3 Sleep stage II. Sleep spindles (hollow arrows), K complexes (filled arrow), and posterior occipital sharp transients of sleep (POSTS) (dashed arrow) are seen.

Table 4.3 Benign variants (no disease significance)

Benign variants	Features
Subclinical rhythmic electrographic discharge in adults (SREDA)	5–7 Hz sharply contoured rhythmic theta waves. More predominant in posterior temporal regions.
Midline theta	Also called "Ciganek rhythm." Rhythmic sinusoidal, arciform activity over electrodes Fz/Cz (midline) with a frequency of 4–7 Hz.
Frontal arousal rhythm	7–10 Hz. Trains of monophasic activity, bifrontal, maximal at electrodes F3/F4.
14 and 6 positive bursts	14 and 6 Hz. Rhythmic positive arciform spikes of 0.5–1-s duration.
Small sharp spikes (SSSs)	Also called "benign epileptiform transients of sleep" (BETS). Less than 50 μV amplitude and less than 50 ms duration. Anterior to midtemporal regions (Fig. 4.4).
6 Hz spike and wave	5–7 Hz. Also called "phantom spike and wave." The spike has a very small amplitude compared to the slow wave (<25 μV).
Wicket spikes	6–11 Hz. Monophasic, arciform, isolated, or in trains. More predominant from anterior to midtemporal regions (Fig. 4.5).
Rhythmic midtemporal discharges (RMTDs)	4–7 Hz. "Psychomotor variant." Train of rhythmic theta activity with variable morphology but often with a notched appearance. It is seen during drowsiness or stage II sleep. It does not evolve in frequency or morphology as focal seizures, so it should not be confused with intermittent slowing over the temporal lobe often seen in patients with temporal lobe epilepsy [8].
Posterior slow waves of youth	Delta waves with superimposed alpha frequencies. In posterior regions. Prominent in ages 3–10 years.
Lambda waves	Biphasic waves with an initial upward deflection followed by a downward phase (Fig. 4.6).

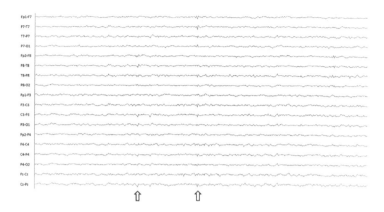

Fig. 4.4 Small sharp spikes (SSSs). Low amplitude (<50 μV) and duration (<50 ms).

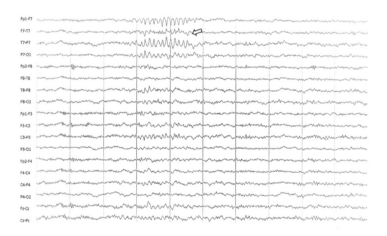

Fig. 4.5 Wicket spikes. 6–11 Hz monophasic, arciform, isolated, or in trains, more predominant from anterior to midtemporal regions.

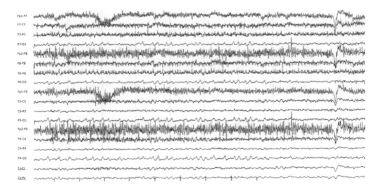

Fig. 4.6 Lambda waves. Biphasic waves with a "λ" shape, best seen over the occipital regions.

What Are Abnormal EEG Findings and Do They All Mean Epilepsy?

INTERICTAL ABNORMALITIES

These abnormalities are seen in EEGs between seizures and can be divided into either epileptiform or nonepileptiform abnormalities.

Epileptiform Abnormalities

Interictal epileptiform abnormalities comprise "sharp waves" or "spikes," are easily differentiated from background activity, and are seen in patients with epilepsy. There are three types:

- Focal epileptiform discharges: These are epileptiform discharges localized to one hemisphere or discrete brain regions and are indicative of focal epilepsy. These are most typically spikes or sharp waves (Fig. 4.7).
- Generalized epileptiform discharges: These are discharges that are synchronous and symmetric in both hemispheres. They typically

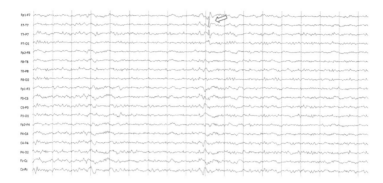

Fig. 4.7 Sharp waves. Sharp waves arising from the left temporal area, maximal at F7.

are spikes/sharp waves and followed by high amplitude slow waves (together called complexes) and most commonly indicate generalized epilepsy. Some specific generalized patterns like 3 Hz spike and wave (childhood absence epilepsy) or 3–4 Hz spike and wave complexes and polyspikes (juvenile myoclonic epilepsy) can indicate more specific syndromic diagnoses (Fig. 4.8).

- Lateralized periodic discharges (LPD): These are discharges that occur repetitively and semiperiodically, typically between 0.5 and 2 Hz in one hemisphere or region. They are commonly observed in the setting of acute/subacute cortical lesions or may indicate a highly epileptogenic focus in patients with seizures. At least 24 hours of video EEG monitoring is often recommended with this EEG finding (Fig. 4.9).

Nonepileptiform Abnormalities

Interictal nonepileptiform abnormalities suggest some degree of brain dysfunction, but they are not indicative of epilepsy. These include:

- Slowing: This term includes EEG activities that are abnormally slow for the age of the patient or state of consciousness.

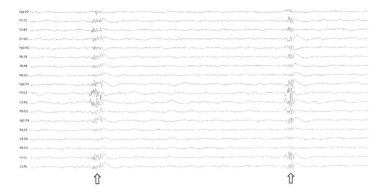

Fig. 4.8 Polyspikes. Generalized polyspikes in a patient with juvenile myoclonic epilepsy.

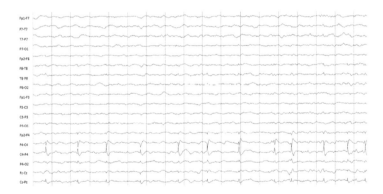

Fig. 4.9 Lateralized periodic discharges (LPDs). Right parasagittal LPD, maximum C4, with a periodic frequency from 0.5 to 1 Hz.

○ Focal slowing: one region or hemisphere is slower than the corresponding contralateral side. Focal slowing indicates focal dysfunction.

- Intermittent focal slowing (<80% of the EEG) can be normal, particularly in drowsiness, and patients over 40 years of age when it is bilateral. However, unilateral slowing is abnormal. If rhythmic and more commonly in the delta range, it can be associated with a higher risk of acute seizures and is called lateralized rhythmic delta activity (LRDA) [9].

- Continuous focal slowing is noted when >80% of the EEG has that slowing and most commonly is interpreted as a structural lesion [10].

○ Generalized slowing: Both hemispheres are slower than expected for age and state of consciousness. Generalized slowing indicates diffuse brain dysfunction (encephalopathy).

- Intermittent generalized slowing (<80% of the EEG) during awake state and not being caused by drowsiness is indicative of a mild encephalopathy.

- Continuous generalized slowing (>80% of the EEG) and not being caused by drowsiness is usually seen with loss of posterior background activity and indicates between a moderate to severe encephalopathy.

- If the slowing amplitude is <10μV, the pattern is called background suppression. In pharmacologically induced comas, there can be a burst suppression with interspersed periods of background suppression interrupted by high amplitude bursts (Fig. 4.10).

- Asymmetry: This term refers to >50% amplitude differences between corresponding contralateral brain regions of EEG activities (e.g., posterior dominant rhythm, sleep spindles). Like slowing, asymmetry indicates a brain lesion in one hemisphere. An additional consideration is a skull defect (i.e., burr hole, craniotomy, etc.)

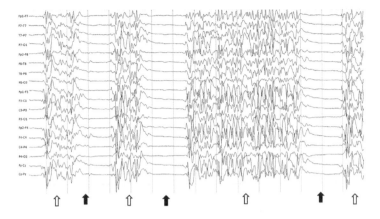

Fig. 4.10 Burst suppression. Low-voltage activity (<10 μV) (black arrows) interrupted by high-amplitude bursts (white arrows).

- ○ Increased voltage is typically seen after burr holes or craniotomies known as breach rhythm, because electrodes record brain electrical activity without increased impediment from the skull.
- ○ Decreased voltage is usually seen due to an increased material interposed between cortex and electrodes (e.g., subdural hemorrhage) [11].
- Generalized periodic patterns (GPDs): These are relatively stereotypical waveforms, which frequently have a periodic repetition rate. A generalized periodic pattern indicates an acute or subacute, severe diffuse encephalopathy, or even brain damage. Some GPDs can indicate diagnoses with modest, although not absolute, specificity. The repetition rate and waveform are relatively characteristic, depending on the origin of the encephalopathy.
  - ○ Triphasic waves are a specific GPD typical of metabolic encephalopathy (Fig. 4.11) [10, 12]
  - ○ Periodic discharges after an anoxic injury are often associated with myoclonic seizures (Fig. 4.12)

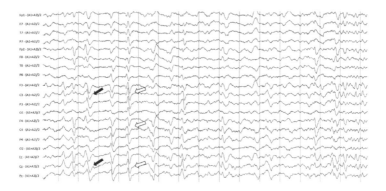

Fig. 4.11 Triphasic waves (also called generalized periodic discharge [GPD] with triphasic morphology). Note the three phases with a frontocentral predominance best visualized at the white arrows: an upward phase I, a downward phase II and again upward phase III. Phase II has the highest voltage. They have an anterior-posterior lag, best noted with black arrows. This is in an ear average referential montage, which can improve triphasic wave appearance.

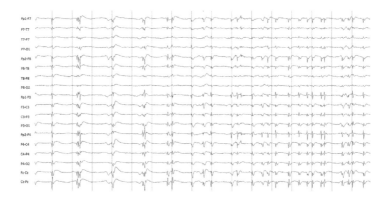

Fig. 4.12 Generalized periodic discharge with spikes. Note the periodic spike/polyspikes with a frequency between 0.5 and 3 Hz. This sample was taken from a patient after cardiac arrest.

- ◦ Periodic discharges recurring every 4 seconds is highly indicative of subacute sclerosing panencephalitis
- ◦ Periodic discharges recurring every 2 seconds is characteristic of adults Creutzfeldt–Jakob disease [10, 11].

Ictal Patterns

- Rhythmic activity: fast (alpha, beta) or slow (delta, theta) rhythmical, often sinusoidal, activity that *evolves* with time in frequency, morphology, amplitude (Fig. 4.13) and/or distribution. Frequency and amplitude of these activities can increase or decrease and can spread to other regions in the same hemisphere or spread to the contralateral side while eventually becoming generalized.
- Repetitive epileptiform discharges (spikes or sharp waves): intermixed with and/or followed by rhythmical activity that evolves over time in frequency, morphology, amplitude, and/or distribution.

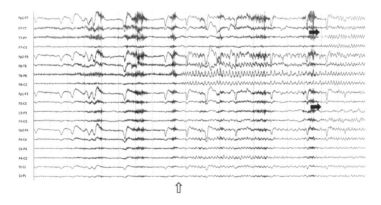

Fig. 4.13 Focal seizure. Abrupt appearance of sharply contoured rhythmic theta activity over the right temporal > parasagittal chains (hollow arrow), evolving in frequency, amplitude, and spreading 8 seconds later to the left hemisphere (black arrows).

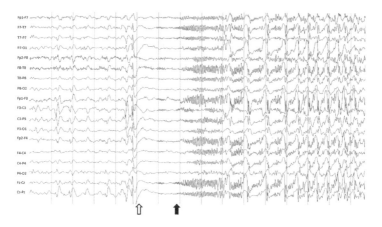

Fig. 4.14 Generalized seizure. Abrupt appearance of electrodecrement (hollow arrow), followed by fast activity (black arrow).

- Electrodecrement (flattening of brain waves or suppression): in one hemisphere or generalized with or without fast frequencies (Fig. 4.14).

The region of the EEG ictal onset helps with the localization of the epileptogenic zone.

- Temporal lobe epilepsy: Most temporal lobe epilepsies have localized EEG findings, seen in 90% of mesial temporal lobe epilepsy and 75% neocortical temporal lobe seizures [13, 14]. A rhythmic theta pattern at onset is highly specific for temporal and less common in extratemporal lobe epilepsies (Fig. 4.13).

- Frontal lobe epilepsy: Particularly from the mesial structures, tend to present with an electrodecrement or generalized EEG onset. More challengingly, only a third of cases have a localized EEG seizure pattern [12].

- Posterior quadrant epilepsy: Shows a localized onset pattern in up to half of the cases [12].

- The ictal pattern in generalized epilepsies (Fig. 4.14) usually mimics the interictal EEG abnormalities:
  - The EEG during typical absence seizures shows the same 2.5–3.5 Hz spike and wave complexes seen interictally
  - The EEG during myoclonic seizures shows a burst of polyspike and wave complexes seen interictally.

How Do I Interpret the EEG Report?

The EEG report is a concise description of the presence or absence of normal findings as well as a description of any abnormalities, whether epileptiform or nonepileptiform. Table 4.4 includes the interpretation of the different findings.

Magnetoencephalography

Magnetoencephalography (MEG) is a complementary tool of EEG. In brief, electricity travels in a straight line while magnetism travels in a circle surrounding that line. In essence, MEG and EEG allow study of the same potential, just from a different plane.

Like EEG, MEG enables localization, characterization of dipole strength and orientation, and estimation of the epileptic zone [15]. Magnetoencephalography is typically performed in patients with DRE in a presurgical evaluation to help localize the epileptogenic zone.

In patients evaluated preoperatively, MEG has an average sensitivity of 70% [16]. Magnetoencephalography measures magnetic currents and it is maximally sensitive to dipoles oriented tangentially to the brain surface, which often corresponds to sulcal activity. The strength of the magnetic field decreases in proportion to the square of the distance from the current dipole, according to the Biot–Savart law. Therefore, the sensitivity of MEG to deep sources is lower [17].

Table 4.4 EEG report interpretation

Pattern		Findings	Interpretation
PDR		Normal (adult 8–13 Hz)	Normal (Fig. 4.1)
		Slow	7–8 Hz: Mild encephalopathy
			6–7 Hz: Moderate encephalopathy
			<6 Hz or absence of PDR: Severe encephalopathy
Photoparoxysmal response		If located in posterior head regions and not sustained beyond photic stimulation end	No clinic relevance
Normal variants			Listed in Table 4.3
Epileptiform	Focal	Spikes	No clinical correlate
		Sharp waves (Fig. 4.7)	Diagnostic for epilepsy
		Spike and wave complexes	
		Polyspikes	
		Benign epileptiform discharges of childhood	Seizure history present: Benign Rolandic epilepsy
			Seizure history absent: Incidental normal finding in some children
	Generalized	3 Hz (2.5–3.5 Hz) spike and wave complexes	Suggestive of genetic/idiopathic epilepsy

	Pattern	Interpretation
	Polyspike wave complexes (Fig. 4.8)	Suggestive of genetic/idiopathic epilepsy
	Slow spike and wave complexes	Suggestive of epileptic encephalopathy (e.g., Lennox–Gastaut syndrome)
	Hypsarrhythmia	Suggestive of epileptic encephalopathy (e.g., West syndrome)
Photoparoxysmal response	If there are generalized discharges, ± sustained beyond photic stimulation end	Likely associated with epilepsy
Nonepileptiform	Background slow	Mild to moderate encephalopathy
	Intermittent slow	Generalized: Mild encephalopathy / Focal: Local dysfunction
	Continuous slow	Generalized: Moderate to severe encephalopathy / Focal: Structural lesion
Other patterns	Excessive fast	Encephalopathy or sedative medication effect
	Asymmetry	Decreased voltage: Structural lesion / Increased voltage: Skull defect
	Periodic pattern	May indicate acute (e.g., anoxic brain injury) or subacute (e.g., Creutzfeldt-Jakob disease) brain damage
	Triphasic waves	Indicative of metabolic encephalopathy

Table 4.4 (cont.)

Pattern	Findings	Interpretation
	Lateralized periodic discharges (Fig. 4.9)	Potentially epileptogenic lesion or acute/subacute cortical injury (e.g., stroke)
	Burst suppression (Fig. 4.10)	Severe diffuse encephalopathy secondary to brain damage or pharmacologically induced coma
	Background suppression	Severe diffuse encephalopathy
		Suggests diffuse brain damage or pharmacologically induced coma
	Alpha coma/stupor	Anoxic or toxic encephalopathy
	Spindle coma/stupor	Anoxic or toxic encephalopathy
	Beta coma/stupor	Anoxic or toxic encephalopathy
	Theta coma/stupor	Nonspecific encephalopathy
	Delta coma/stupor	Anoxic or toxic encephalopathy
	Electrocerebral inactivity	Severe brain damage, may indicate brain death

This chapter is intended as a brief, practical overview for understanding the utility of different EEG types as well as understanding basic EEG findings and reports. For comprehensive review, the authors suggest an excellent free EEG text and atlas for comprehensive evaluation of this subject made available by the American Epilepsy Society [18].

Works Cited

1. DB Burkholder, JW Britton, V Rajasekaran et al. Routine vs extended outpatient EEG for the detection of interictal epileptiform discharges. *Neurology*. 2016;86(16):1524–30.

2. M Salinsky, R Kanter, and RM Dasheiff. Effectiveness of multiple EEGs in supporting the diagnosis of epilepsy: An operational curve. *Epilepsia*. 1987;28(4):331–4.

3. CA Marsan and LSZivin. Factors related to the occurrence of typical paroxysmal abnormalities in the EEG records of epileptic patients. *Epilepsia*. 1970;11(4):361–81.

4. MA King, MR Newton, GD Jackson et al. Epileptology of the first-seizure presentation: A clinical, electroencephalographic, and magnetic resonance imaging study of 300 consecutive patients. *Lancet*. 1998;352(9133):1007–11.

5. JR Daube and DI Rubin. *Clinical Neurophysiology*. 3rd ed. New York: Oxford University Press; 2009. xxvii.

6. CS Nayak and AC Anilkumar. *EEG Normal Waveforms*. Treasure Island, FL: StatPearls; 2021.

7. V Rey, S Aybek, M Maeder-Ingvar, and AO Rossetti. Positive occipital sharp transients of sleep (POSTS): A reappraisal. *Clin Neurophysiol*. 2009;120(3):472–5.

8. H Lüders and S Noachtar. *Atlas and Classification of Electroencephalography*. Philadelphia: Saunders; 2000. xiv.

9. P Salvioni Chiabotti, A Vicino, and AO Rossetti. Lateralized rhythmic delta activity: A peri-ictal feature beyond epilepsy. *Clin Neurophysiol*. 2021;132(6):1302–3.

10. S Shorvon, R Guerrini, M Cook, and S Lhatoo. *Oxford Textbook of Epilepsy and Epileptic Seizures*. Oxford: Oxford University Press; 2013.

11. LJ Hirsch, MWK Fong, M Leitinger et al. American Clinical Neurophysiology Society's standardized critical care EEG terminology: 2021 version. *J Clin Neurophysiol*. 2021;38(1):1–29.

12. N Foldvary, G Klem, J Hammel et al. The localizing value of ictal EEG in focal epilepsy. *Neurology*. 2001;57(11):2022–8.

13. M Javidan. Electroencephalography in mesial temporal lobe epilepsy: A review. *Epilepsy Res Treat.* 2012;2012:637430.

14. SK Lee, SY Lee, KK Kim et al. Surgical outcome and prognostic factors of cryptogenic neocortical epilepsy. *Ann Neurol.* 2005;58(4):525–32.

15. S Murakami and Y Okada. Contributions of principal neocortical neurons to magnetoencephalography and electroencephalography signals. *J Physiol.* 2006;575(pt. 3):925–36.

16. H Stefan, C Hummel, G Scheler et al. Magnetic brain source imaging of focal epileptic activity: A synopsis of 455 cases. *Brain.* 2003;126(pt. 11):2396–405.

17. J Malmivuo, V Suihko, and H Eskola. Sensitivity distributions of EEG and MEG measurements. *IEEE Trans Biomed Eng.* 1997;44(3):196–208.

18. EK St. Louis and LC Frey. *Electroencephalography: An Introductory Text and Atlas of Normal and Abnormal Findings in Adults, Children, and Infants.* Chicago: American Epilepsy Society; 2016. www.ncbi.nlm.nih.gov/books/NBK390354/pdf/Bookshelf_NBK390354.pdf.

5

What Are Common Epilepsy Imaging Findings in New Onset and Chronic Epilepsy Care?

Ordering an Epilepsy Protocol MRI for Your Patient

The International League Against Epilepsy (ILAE) Neuroimaging Task Force recommends a brain magnetic resonance imaging (MRI) be obtained after the first seizure. This MRI can potentially identify seizure etiology and its impact on recurrence risk. These data in turn impact clinical management [1]. Moreover, in new onset epilepsy patients with an MRI identifying a clear etiology, referral to an epilepsy surgery center can be considered for definitive therapy.

To maximize MRI yield, the ILAE Neuroimaging Task Force defined a minimum set of MRI sequences, known as Harmonized Neuroimaging of Epilepsy Structural Sequences (HARNESS-MRI) protocol, that applies to both children and adults [1, 2]. The ILAE Neuroimaging Task force recommends obtaining an MRI with HARNESS protocol, even if previous MRIs are normal. The *mandatory sequences* of the HARNESS-MRI protocol, preferentially on a 3 Tesla (3T) MRI include the following.

- High-resolution 3D T1-weighted MRI
  - Clear depiction of brain anatomy and morphology
  - Advantages: Optimal to evaluate gray/white matter differentiation as well as gray matter thickness and gyration
  - Disadvantages: Not sensitive for certain pathologies like hippocampal sclerosis (HS).

- High-resolution 3D fluid-attenuated inversion recovery (FLAIR)
  - Evaluation of signal anomalies.
  - Advantages: Improved visualization of hyperintense cortical lesions due to CSF attenuation
  - Disadvantages: May not detect subtle HS or pathology, particularly before age 24 months since myelination is incomplete.
- High in-plane resolution 2D coronal T2-weighted MRI
  - Optimal visualization of hippocampal internal structure
  - Advantages: Facilitates diagnosis of HS
  - Disadvantages: CSF hyperintensity can obscure cortical lesions.

The following *optional sequences* of the HARNESS protocol should be included if certain pathologies are suspected:

- Gadolinium-enhanced 3D T1-weighted MRI
  - Evaluation of tumors, vascular malformations, or intracranial infections
- Susceptibility-weighted imaging (SWI) and gradient echo (GRE) 3D T2-weighted MRI
  - Evaluation of calcifications, blood products, and iron deposits

Of note, the HARNESS-MRI protocol is defined for both 1.5T and 3T MR scanners in an attempt to account for economic differences among territories. However, overall spatial resolution may be inferior with 1.5T. In a retrospective review of unselected patients who had a brain MRI at 1.5T and subsequently at 3T, 5% of the patients were found to have new clinically relevant new diagnoses [3].

7T MR scanners are newly approved by the FDA in clinical practice. They can improve visualization, characterization, and delineation of brain lesions. Therefore, 7T MRI scans may be indicated for patients with drug-resistant epilepsy for either "lesion negative MRI" or 3T MRI with equivocal findings. This may improve detection and visualization of potentially epileptogenic lesions [4]. However, further studies are needed to assess the impact of 7T MRI results on surgical outcome [5].

What Are the Most Common Inpatient Imaging Findings?

BRAIN HEMORRHAGES

Brain hemorrhages can appear differently at different time points given evolving hemoglobin degradation. When acute intracranial hemorrhage is suspected, a brain computer tomography (CT) is the imaging of choice.

Computer Tomography

Blood collections in the acute phase appear hyperdense (white) on CT. Over time, blood hyper density signals progressively decrease on CT as the blood resorbs. Once blood is completely reabsorbed, it appears as a focal hypodense (dark) area with cerebral atrophy and possible local ventricular dilation, also known as ex vacuo dilatation.

Magnetic Resonance Imaging

Blood products are seen as focal hypointensities (dark) on SWI and GRE T2-weighted sequences. The hemorrhage appearance on T1 and T2 sequences over time is summarized in Table 5.1.

Table 5.1 Appearance of blood based on time and MRI sequence		
Timing	T1	T2
Hyperacute (0–24 hours)	Isointense	Hyperintense
Acute (24–72 hours)	Isointense	Hypointense
Early subacute (72 hours–7 days)	Hyperintense	Hypointense
Late subacute (7–14 days)	Hyperintense	Hyperintense
Chronic (>14 days)	Hypointense	Hypointense
Note: Hyperintense is bright and hypointense is dark on MRI		

GLIOMAS

Radiologic evaluation of tumor should define the location and number of tumor(s). Subsequent studies should specifically note stability and progression overtime. Moreover, it is critical to compare subsequent studies to the initial study. When comparing consecutive scans only, tumor growth may be missed due to inherent slow progression for low-grade gliomas. The Brain Tumor Imaging Protocol notes brain MRI should include the following sequences at a minimum power of 1.5T [6]:

(1) Pre- and postcontrast 3D T1-weighted MRI
   ○ Again, T1 sequences provide optimal anatomic definition
   ○ Precontrast hyperintensity (bright) is seen in lesions containing hemoglobin degradation products, fat, melanin, minerals, and high content in proteins [7]
   ○ Postcontrast enhancement (bright) demonstrates disruption of the blood–brain barrier and can be commonly interpreted as tumor invasion with an accompanying lesion
   ○ Of note, imaging acquisition should not start earlier than 2–5 minutes after contrast administration. Otherwise, tumoral lesions may be missed.

(2) Axial T2 FLAIR and axial T2-weighted MRI
   ○ Hyperintensity (bright) is seen in vasogenic and infiltrative edema and gliosis.

(3) Axial DWI
   ○ Hyperintensity (bright) is seen with cytotoxic edema.

Other techniques can be used to further characterize tumor type and to aid surgical planning:

(1) Magnetic resonance spectroscopy (MRS)
   ○ Analysis of creatine (normal cellular metabolism), choline (Cho, cell membrane turnover), N-acetyl aspartate (NAA, neuronal viability), myo-inositol (MI, astrocyte integrity), lipid (necrosis), and lactate (hypoxia).

(2) Perfusion
  ○ Provides information about relative blood volume and flow in one brain area compared to neighboring regions.
(3) Diffusion tensor imaging (DTI)
  ○ Assessment of white matter tracts.
(4) Functional MRI (fMRI) is discussed later in this chapter.

While brain MRI is essential in tumor care, no definitive diagnostic radiological features exist for any one tumor type. Therefore, an accurate differential diagnosis of the histological tumor type requires additional clinical information, such as the age, symptom duration, presence of an extracranial primary malignancy, and history of prior brain insults, particularly radiotherapy [6].

As a rule of thumb, high-grade gliomas appear hyperintense on T2/FLAIR, typically exhibit heterogeneous postcontrast enhancement, have high Cho peaks on MRS, and show increased blood flow and volume on perfusion techniques [6]. Table 5.2 highlights distinctive clinical and radiological features of the habitual glioma types [8].

BRAIN METASTASES

Brain metastases are the most common intracranial neoplasm in adults. They occur supratentorially 80% of the time, often at the gray–white matter junction. They less commonly involve the cerebellum (15%) or brainstem (5%). Abdominal and pelvic cancers more commonly metastasize to the posterior fossa [8].

Radiological features:
(1) Postcontrast imaging shows a ring appearance
  ○ Of note, metastasis enhance several minutes after contrast injection. Therefore, immediate postcontrast imaging (i.e., CT angiography) is substandard for metastasis assessment.
(2) Multifocal far more frequently (60–75%) in contrast to glioblastoma

Table 5.2 Imaging characteristics of select primary brain tumors

	Glioblastoma	Diffuse astrocytoma	Oligodendroglioma
Peak age (years)	45–70	30–50	25–45
Habitual location	Subcortical hemispheric white matter	Subcortical hemispheric white matter	Cortical
Enhancement	Ring-like pattern with irregular walls, due to central necrosis	Variable	Variable. Minimal patchy or lacy enhancement can be seen in up to 50% of cases
Hemorrhage	Common	Rare	Rare
Calcification	Rare, thought to be secondary to preexisting low-grade glioma	Rare	Common
MRS	↑ Cho, lactate, lipids ↓ NAA, MI	↑ Cho, MI ↓ NAA	↑ Cho ↓ NAA
Other characteristics	Significant peritumoral edema with mass effect. Can infiltrate the contralateral hemisphere through white matter tracts, giving a "butterfly" appearance. Typically solitary; multifocal or in <1% of cases	Peritumoral edema is uncommon	Peritumoral edema is uncommon

(3) Vasogenic edema typically extends into white matter in a "finger" pattern

(4) Central necrosis (heterogenous enhancement and FLAIR signal) can be a feature

(5) Calcifications are rare except with either indolent metastasis or prior irradiation

(6) Melanoma and small cell lung carcinoma have the highest rate of multifocal metastasis and concomitant hemorrhage

(7) Magnetic resonance spectroscopy show low or absent NAA given the lack of neuroglial elements

(8) Subcortical white matter is displaced on DTI. In contrast, high-grade gliomas disrupt or invade white matter tracts due to its primary evolution from brain.

What Are the Most Common Outpatient Imaging Findings?

HIPPOCAMPAL SCLEROSIS

Hippocampal sclerosis is radiologically defined by these hippocampus changes (Fig. 5.1):

(1) Volume loss

(2) Internal architecture loss

(3) T2/FLAIR hyperintensity (bright)

(4) Decreased T1 signal intensity (dark) [2, 9, 10].

Other MRI findings include temporal lobe atrophy, temporal horn dilation, blurring of the gray–white interphase of the anterior temporal lobe, and volume loss of the amygdala and entorhinal cortex, among others [11, 12].

Of note, a normal variant is *hippocampal malrotation*. This can be seen in healthy subjects as well as temporal lobe epilepsy patients.

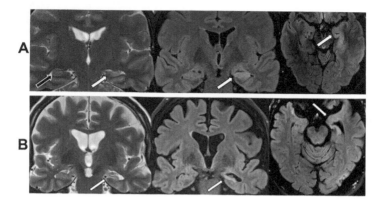

Fig. 5.1 Left HS. Coronal T2 (left), and coronal (central) and axial (right) T2 FLAIR sequences. In both (A) and (B) there is decreased size of the head and body of the left hippocampus (white arrow). In addition, the left hippocampus shows a hyperintense FLAIR signal. (A) shows earlier left HS; note normal right hippocampus internal architecture (black arrow). (B) shows a more advanced stage of left HS (white arrow) in a different patient. The hippocampus is substantially atrophied with prominent left ventricular horn asymmetry.

Hippocampal malrotation is characterized by an abnormally round, vertically oriented hippocampus with a deep collateral sulcus and it is considered an anatomic variant [13].

Postprocessing can quantify hippocampal volume and signal changes. This may detect subtle atrophy and signal changes unseen by visual inspection alone.

ENCEPHALOCELES

Encephaloceles are herniations of the brain parenchyma through the skull and meninges. These can be congenital or occur after traumatic brain injuries. Encephaloceles have been recently recognized as an etiology for epilepsy, particularly temporal lobe epilepsy [14, 15]. These

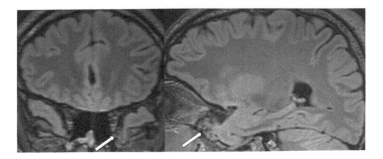

Fig. 5.2 Anteromesial temporal encephalocele (arrow) seen in FLAIR coronal (left) and FLAIR sagittal (right) planes. Note the extension of cerebrum past the skull boundary and varied appearance based on plane of view.

are typically found along the greater wing of the sphenoidal bone, which causes the adjacent temporal lobe to poke through the skull defect [16].

Encephaloceles can be seen on MRI as protrusions of gray matter with or without signal changes, best noted on T2/FLAIR (Fig. 5.2). They are associated with MRI features of idiopathic intracranial hypertension including flattening of the posterior globe of the eye, prominent CSF space around the optic nerve, empty sella turcica, and an enlarged Meckel cave [16]. Temporal encephalocele detection can be improved by using 3T MRI showing an increase in signal in T2 sequences and FLAIR, combined with a high-resolution CT to demonstrate the skull defects.

LONG-TERM EPILEPSY-ASSOCIATED TUMORS

Any brain tumor type, whether malignant or benign, that involves cortex can lead to epilepsy. Still, a subset of low-grade tumors from a broad different histopathological spectrum are notoriously associated with epilepsy. These have been grouped under the concept of long-term epilepsy-associated tumors (LEATs). The two most common types are the following [17].

- *Gangliogliomas* are frequently associated with epilepsy. The most common location is the temporal lobe, although they can be in any lobe, most commonly in the peripheral part of cortex. The combination of solid, cystic, and calcium components gives the aspect of a heterogeneous lesion on MRI, with little mass effect and vasogenic edema. Susceptibility-weighted imaging T2-weighted images in addition to CT facilitate visualization of calcifications. Gangliogliomas can variably enhance in nodular or linear patterns. There can be associated focal leptomeningeal enhancement as well. Magnetic resonance spectroscopy shows a decrease in the Cho/creatine and NAA/creatine ratios, with an increased Cho/NAA ratio (Fig. 5.3).

- *Desembryoplastic neuroepithelial tumors (DNETs)* are the most epileptogenic neoplasm. The most frequent location is the temporal

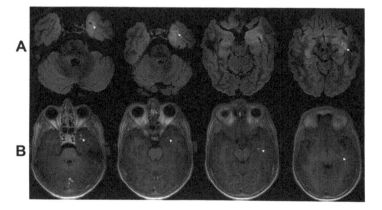

Fig. 5.3 Left temporal ganglioglioma. Axial T2 FLAIR (A) shows a hyperintense lesion, extending from the left anterior temporal pole to the left mesial temporal lobe, involving both the cortex and subcortical white matter, containing multiple cystic components (white arrow). Note expansion of the cortex, most evident in the region of the amygdala (label). Axial T1 postcontrast administration (B) shows two separate irregularly shaped enhancing components along the anterior and posterior margins (arrowhead).

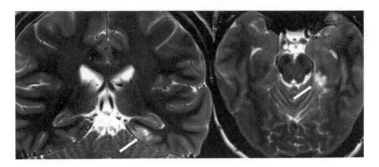

Fig. 5.4 Left parahippocampal DNET presented with T2-weighted coronal (left) and axial (right) images. Note the cystic appearance (arrow), often referred to as "bubbly."

lobe. These are well-defined lesions that characteristically do not grow. They can have a cystic or multicystic appearance and can contain calcifications. Contrast enhancement is seen in about 30% of the cases. Magnetic resonance spectroscopy is most commonly normal (Fig. 5.4).

LEATs may be associated with coexistent HS or with surrounding dysplastic tissue (FCD type IIIb).

BRAIN CAVERNOMAS

Brain cavernomas are vascular malformations consisting of thin endothelium lacking elastic and muscular layers. Cavernomas' thin walls predispose to leakage of blood, producing hemosiderin deposits and gliosis in surrounding cortical tissue.

Cavernomas are multilobulated lesions containing blood products at different stages. Table 5.1 shows the varying appearance based on sequence and time.

Gradient echo-T2 sequences and SWI increase the radiologic sensitivity of cavernoma diagnosis (Fig. 5.5). These sequences can show a hemosiderin rim, considered the epileptogenic feature of cavernomas.

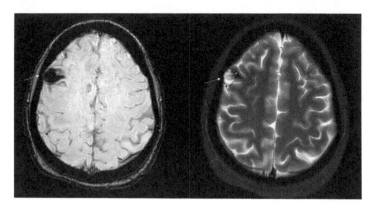

Fig. 5.5 Cavernoma. Susceptibility-weighted imaging (left) and T2 (right) sequences. Lobulated heterogeneously T2 hyperintense hemosiderin rimmed lesion in the right middle frontal gyrus periphery with hemosiderin extending medially, without surrounding edema.

Cavernomas do not exhibit significant contrast enhancement, mass effect, or edema, except in the setting of an acute/recent hemorrhage [18]. Contrasted imaging is recommended presurgically to evaluate potential adjacent developmental venous anomalies that may influence the surgical approach.

Since cavernomas are dynamic processes that may grow and can periodically bleed, follow-up imaging is recommended, initially at 6 months and yearly thereafter. With acute neurological change, repeat imaging should be sought urgently [18].

FOCAL CORTICAL DYSPLASIAS

Focal cortical dysplasias (FCDs) are a heterogeneous group of malformations of cortical development (MCD) characterized by cortical dyslamination with or without dysmorphic neurons. Focal cortical dysplasias are classified into three different types with a detailed histopathological discussion beyond the scope of this manual [19].

Focal cortical dysplasias are identified by focal cortical thickening, gray–white matter differentiation loss, focal volume loss, and focal T2/FLAIR hyperintensities. Focal cortical dysplasia type IIb is best noted by MRI and characterized by the *transmantle sign*, a hyperintense T2/FLAIR signal extending from the cortex to the ipsilateral lateral ventricle (Fig. 5.6). This tract is the visualization of the abnormal cortical migration that resulted in the FCD formation. At times, the hyperintense signal of an FCD is only noted in the bottom of the sulcus [2].

Unfortunately, MRI findings in FCD types I and IIa are often subtle and escape visual detection. To facilitate FCD detection, postprocessing techniques and quantitative MRI analyses can be performed where available [20].

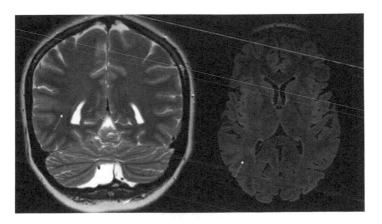

Fig. 5.6 Focal cortical dysplasia type IIb. Coronal T2 (left) and axial T2 FLAIR (right). Band of T2 hyperintensity (arrow) extending from the ventricular margin to the surface of the right temporoparietal junction, known as transmantle sign. Histopathology confirmed the FCD type IIb radiologic diagnosis.

HETEROTOPIAS

Heterotopias are a second MCD type that result from abnormal neuronal migration from the subependymal to the cortical plate [21]. More plainly said, heterotopias are abnormally located gray matter. Depending on the stage in which the disruption of migration occurs, different arrangements of gray matter can be seen: subependymal, subcortical, and band heterotopia [21, 22].

- *Periventricular nodular heterotopia (PVNH)* is the most common heterotopia type. Periventricular nodular heterotopia are visualized as round/ovoid subependymal nodules of gray matter in the periventricular region protruding into the ventricle. Nodules can be single or multiple (Fig. 5.7) and do not enhance with contrast. The most common location is the trigon and occipital horns of lateral ventricles. Cortex overlying the nodules may be dysplastic.

- *Subcortical heterotopia* are bands of gray matter within hemispheric white matter. It can be further classified as *nodular* if there is no

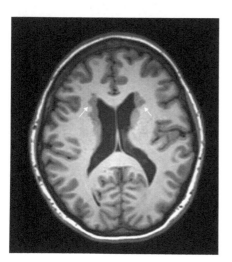

Fig. 5.7 Bilateral PVNH on T1. Note the presence of subependymal nodules lining the lateral walls of the lateral ventricles. These nodules are isointense to normal cortical gray matter.

definite continuity with the cerebral cortex, or *curvilinear*, when it is continuous with the cortex and has appearance of an enfolded cortex. A combination of both patterns can be seen in the same patient.

- *Band heterotopia (aka double cortex)* appears as smooth bilateral bands of gray matter in the white matter in between the cerebral cortex and the ventricular surface.

All heterotopia types can be seen with other MCDs including FCD, polymicrogyria (PMG), pachygyria, and lissencephaly [21].

POLYMICROGYRIA

Polymicrogyria is an MCD resulting from abnormal postmigrational development [21]. This gives cortex an excessively folded or stippled appearance with fusion of adjacent gyri and shallow sulci. The most common location of PMG is in the perisylvian region (Fig. 5.8).

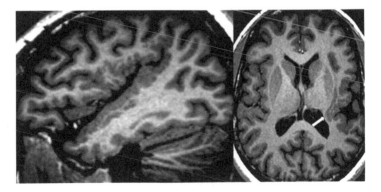

Fig. 5.8 Left perisylvian polymicrogyria shown with T1 sagittal (left) and axial (right) images. Note the extensive involvement of the perisylvian tissue, most notable in the posterior portion. This patient also has a curvilinear band heterotopia (arrow) seen on the axial image.

Polymicrogyria appearance on MRI changes with a patient's age due to changes in myelination. In newborns and young infants, in whom myelination is incomplete, PMG is noted as small, fine undulating cortex with normal thickness on T2-weighted images. After 2 years of age, once myelination is complete, PMG can be detected on T1, T2, and FLAIR MRI sequences by the presence of an abnormal gyral pattern, with an apparent increase in cortical thickness and an irregular cortical–white matter junction because of the microgyria [23].

Other Imaging Topics in Epilepsy Care

A NOTE ON THE USE OF CT IN THE OUTPATIENT SETTING

The role of brain CT is mainly limited to the acute setting, given the better resolution of the images obtained with brain MRI when compared to those of brain CT. A noncontrast CT is the initial imaging of choice in patients presenting with a first seizure in the emergency setting in order to assess pathology that is potentially life threatening and that may require immediate intervention, such as hemorrhages and brain masses. In addition, intravenous contrast may be indicated if there is suspicion for central nervous system infection or small neoplasms and brain MRI is not readily available [1]. Finally, brain perfusion CT (PCT) may help to differentiate an ongoing or recently resolved status epilepticus (regional hyperperfusion) from postictal state or a simultaneous acute ischemic stroke (regional hypoperfusion) [24, 25].

In the outpatient setting, a brain CT is rarely needed if a brain MRI is available. However, a brain CT may be helpful to evaluate skull base defects if a temporal encephalocele is suspected as well as to assess calcified lesions.

FUNCTIONAL IMAGING

18 Fluorodeoxyglucose Positron Emission Tomography

The goal of positron emission tomography (PET) is to detect areas of hypometabolism, which are indicative of focal dysfunction that can correlate with areas involved in seizure generation. Hypometabolism is detected by injection of radiolabeled glucose. The brain area with impaired metabolism takes up less of the radiolabeled glucose and thus does not demonstrate the same level of metabolism compared to the homologous contralateral brain region as well as surrounding ipsilateral brain regions (Fig. 5.9). This concept is also called the *functional deficit zone*, defined as the area or areas of the cortex that are functionally abnormal in between seizures [26].

18 fluorodeoxyglucose PET (18-FDG PET) is not routinely performed in all patients with epilepsy and its indications are mainly reserved for those patients with drug-resistant epilepsy as part of the presurgical work-up, under the following situations:

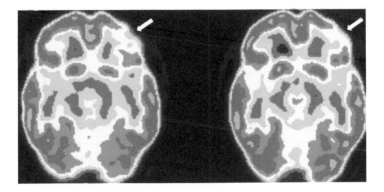

Fig. 5.9 Interictal PET scan demonstrating left frontal hypometabolism (arrow). This hypometabolism correlated with a previously unrecognized focal cortical dysplasia type IIb on MRI.

(1) A brain MRI fails to demonstrate an epileptogenic lesion
(2) There is conflicting data regarding epilepsy localization or lateralization.

While the interictal period looks for PET hypometabolism, it can be useful for localizing status epilepticus if clinical or electroencephalogram (EEG) data are equivocal by showing areas of hypermetabolism [27]. As a corollary, as the uptake pattern in the interictal 18-FDG PET can be affected by an ongoing subclinical seizure, EEG recording before and during the acquisition is recommended if available.

Single Photon Emission Computed Tomography

Single photon emission computed tomography (SPECT) is a functional imaging modality that assesses regional cerebral blood flow (rCBF). The rCBF is used as a correlate of neuronal activity intensity. If performed appropriately early during a seizure, ictal SPECT provides localizing information for the *seizure onset zone* [26]. Early injection time (less than 20 seconds) is critical for the accuracy of ictal SPECT, as later injections may not accurately capture the seizure onset zone. Instead, longer injection times may provide false or nonlocalizing results due to seizure spread. Therefore, seizures of extratemporal origin should last at least 10–15 seconds after ictal SPECT injection so that they may provide truly localizing information.

In order to achieve good injection times, live continuous video-EEG monitoring is required with nursing staff at the bedside ready to inject the tracer via an indwelling intravenous cannula as soon as the first clinical or EEG change is noted. It is important to relate the time of seizure onset to the time of injection so that the ictal SPECT may be accurately interpreted. In addition, the patient's habitual seizure semiology should be confirmed. Single photon emission computed tomography images are usually acquired 10 minutes to 6 hours after injection. One of the main limitations for ictal SPECT is that the test is run only during daytime working hours in most centers. Capturing a seizure in such a limited time frame can be challenging, particularly for patients with nocturnal seizures. Reversing the patient's sleep/wake cycle can be successful, albeit difficult for the patient.

Interpretation of ictal SPECT is optimized by acquisition of a baseline (interictal) SPECT scan. Both SPECT scans are normalized to adjust for dose differences between the ictal and interictal studies. By substraction analysis, areas of hyperperfusion are identified and coregistered to the patient's MRI (technique aka SISCOM [substraction ictal single-photon emission CT coregistered to MRI]) for anatomical interpretation [28]. Concordance of SISCOM focus with the site of surgery is predictive of a seizure improvement after epilepsy surgery, with excellent outcomes in those patients with extratemporal lobe epilepsy and complete resection of the SISCOM focus [29, 30].

Similarly to 18 FDG-PET, the use of SPECT is considered for MRI normal patients or patients whose presurgical evaluation has conflicting data. There is discrepancy among studies comparing the sensitivity of SPECT and 18-FDG PET. This disparity is most likely due to inconsistencies in the SPECT injection time. A study using intracranial EEG results found SPECT injection times within 30 seconds from seizure onset had an 87% sensitivity compared to 56% sensitivity for interictal 18-FDG PET. Nonetheless, there was no effect of imaging concordance and surgical outcome [31].

Functional MRI

Functional MRI assesses focal changes in brain flow by analyzing difference in magnetic properties between oxygenated and deoxygenated hemoglobin, a technique known as blood (BOLD). This is possible due to "neurovascular coupling" principle: focal increases in neuronal activity produce focal increases in cerebral blow flow. The analysis of focal changes in BOLD signal while the patient is performing specific tasks can be used for localization of language, primary motor, primary somatosensory, and visual cortex. This information may be used for

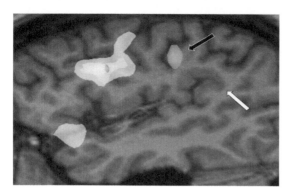

Fig. 5.10 Functional MRI showing language and motor areas. The upper white region depicts Broca's area with the lower white area being artifactual. The gray area (black arrow) depicts lip motor area. The white arrow points to a posterior perisylvian focal cortical dysplasia in close proximity to the lip motor area.

delineating the surgical approach and to assess potential postoperative functional deficits (Fig. 5.10).

During an fMRI, standardized protocols are presented to the patient, depending on the function under investigation. For instance, primary motor cortex can be identified by asking the patient to perform foot- or finger-tapping tasks. Somatosensory function can be assessed performing tactile stimuli by the examiner. For language testing, the patients are given several paradigms that produce language production or comprehension. Finally, visual function can also be assessed by intermittently showing checkerboards to the patient, alternating with blank screens [32].

According to American Academy of Neurology guidelines, fMRI can be considered as a replacement for the Wada test (also called intracarotid amobarbital procedure) for language lateralization in patients with mesial temporal lobe epilepsy, temporal lobe epilepsy in general, or extratemporal epilepsy. However, there is insufficient data for patients with temporal neocortical epilepsy or temporal tumors. Functional MRI can also replace Wada testing in patients with mesial temporal epilepsy for lateralizing memory function but this indication is unclear for other epilepsy types. Lastly, fMRI may be considered to predict postsurgical language deficits after anterior temporal lobe resection as well as visuospatial and verbal memory outcomes [33].

While not widely available, fMRI can also be used to localize regional metabolic changes associated with interictal epileptiform discharges when performed simultaneously with scalp EEG recordings (EEG–fMRI). This information may be helpful to define the source localization hypothesis [34].

Works Cited

1. A Bernasconi, F Cendes, WH Theodore et al. Recommendations for the use of structural magnetic resonance imaging in the care of patients with epilepsy: A consensus report from the International League Against Epilepsy Neuroimaging Task Force. *Epilepsia*. 2019;60(6):1054–68.

2. I Wang, A Bernasconi, B Bernhardt et al. MRI essentials in epileptology: A review from the ILAE Imaging Taskforce. *Epileptic Disord*. 2020;22(4):421–37.

3. GP Winston, C Micallef, BE Kendell et al. The value of repeat neuroimaging for epilepsy at a tertiary referral centre: 16 years of experience. *Epilepsy Res*. 2013;105(3):349–55.

4. G Opheim, A van der Kolk, K Markenroth Bloch et al. 7T Epilepsy Task Force Consensus recommendations on the use of 7T MRI in clinical practice. *Neurology*. 2021;96(7):327–41.

5. R van Lanen, AJ Colon, CJ Wiggins et al. Ultra-high field magnetic resonance imaging in human epilepsy: A systematic review. *Neuroimage Clin*. 2021;30:102602.

6. JE Villanueva-Meyer, MC Mabray, and S Cha. Current clinical brain tumor imaging. *Neurosurgery*. 2017;81(3):397–415.

7. A Zimny, L Zinska, J Bladowska, M Neska-Matuszewska, and M Sasiadek. Intracranial lesions with high signal intensity on T1-weighted MR images: Review of pathologies. *Pol J Radiol*. 2013;78(4):36–46.

8. HB Newton. *Handbook of Neuro-oncology Neuroimaging*. 2nd ed. Cambridge, MA: Academic Press; 2016. xxi.

9. R Kuzniecky, V de la Sayette, R Ethier et al. Magnetic resonance imaging in temporal lobe epilepsy: Pathological correlations. *Ann Neurol*. 1987;22(3):341–7.

10. FG Woermann, GJ Barker, KD Birnie, HJ Meencke, and JS Duncan. Regional changes in hippocampal T2 relaxation and volume: a quantitative magnetic resonance imaging study of hippocampal sclerosis. *J Neurol Neurosurg Psychiatry.* 1998;65(5):656–64.

11. N Bernasconi, J Natsume, and A Bernasconi. Progression in temporal lobe epilepsy: Differential atrophy in mesial temporal structures. *Neurology.* 2005;65(2):223–8.

12. NF Moran, L Lemieux, ND Kitchen, DR Fish, and SD Shorvon. Extrahippocampal temporal lobe atrophy in temporal lobe epilepsy and mesial temporal sclerosis. *Brain.* 2001;124(pt. 1):167–75.

13. MH Tsai, DN Vaughan, Y Perchyonok et al. Hippocampal malrotation is an anatomic variant and has no clinical significance in MRI-negative temporal lobe epilepsy. *Epilepsia.* 2016;57(10):1719–28.

14. A Abou-Hamden, M Lau, G Fabinyi et al. Small temporal pole encephaloceles: A treatable cause of "lesion negative" temporal lobe epilepsy. *Epilepsia.* 2010;51(10):2199–202.

15. T Saavalainen, L Jutila, E Mervaala et al. Temporal anteroinferior encephalocele: An underrecognized etiology of temporal lobe epilepsy? *Neurology.* 2015;85(17):1467–74.

16. ZM Campbell, JM Hyer, S Lauzon et al. Detection and characteristics of temporal encephaloceles in patients with refractory epilepsy. *AJNR Am J Neuroradiol.* 2018;39(8):1468–72.

17. M Giulioni, G Marucci, M Martinoni et al. Epilepsy associated tumors: Review article. *World J Clin Cases.* 2014;2(11):623–41.

18. F Rosenow, MA Alonso-Vanegas, C Baumgartner et al. Cavernoma-related epilepsy: Review and recommendations for management: Report of the Surgical Task Force of the ILAE Commission on Therapeutic Strategies. *Epilepsia.* 2013;54(12):2025–35.

19. I Blumcke, M Thom, E Aronica et al. The clinicopathologic spectrum of focal cortical dysplasias: A consensus classification proposed by an ad hoc Task Force of the ILAE Diagnostic Methods Commission. *Epilepsia.* 2011;52(1):158–74.

20. JS Duncan, GP Winston, MJ Koepp, and S Ourselin. Brain imaging in the assessment for epilepsy surgery. *Lancet Neurol.* 2016;15(4):420–33.

21. AJ Barkovich, R Guerrini, RI Kuzniecky, GD Jackson, and WB Dobyns. A developmental and genetic classification for malformations of cortical development: Update 2012. *Brain.* 2012;135(pt. 5):1348–69.

22. RH Donkol, KM Moghazy, and A Abolenin. Assessment of gray matter heterotopia by magnetic resonance imaging. *World J Radiol.* 2012;4(3):90–6.

23. J Takanashi and AJ Barkovich. The changing MR imaging appearance of polymicrogyria: A consequence of myelination. *Am J Neuroradiol.* 2003;24(5):788–93.

24. D Strambo, V Rey, AO Rossetti et al. Perfusion-CT imaging in epileptic seizures. *J Neurol*. 2018;265(12):2972-9.

25. M Gonzalez-Cuevas, P Coscojuela, E Santamarina et al. Usefulness of brain perfusion CT in focal-onset status epilepticus. *Epilepsia*. 2019;60(7):1317-24.

26. F Rosenow and H Lüders. Presurgical evaluation of epilepsy. *Brain*. 2001;124(pt. 9):1683-700.

27. F Siclari, JO Prior, and AO Rossetti. Ictal cerebral positron emission tomography (PET) in focal status epilepticus. *Epilepsy Res*. 2013;105(3):356-61.

28. W van Paesschen. Ictal SPECT. *Epilepsia*. 2004;45(suppl. 4):35-40.

29. TJ O'Brien, EL So, BP Mullan et al. Subtraction ictal SPECT co-registered to MRI improves clinical usefulness of SPECT in localizing the surgical seizure focus. *Neurology*. 1998;50(2):445-54.

30. TJ O'Brien, EL So, BP Mullan et al. Subtraction peri-ictal SPECT is predictive of extratemporal epilepsy surgery outcome. *Neurology*. 2000;55(11):1668-77.

31. A Desai, K Bekelis, VM Thadani et al. Interictal PET and ictal subtraction SPECT: Sensitivity in the detection of seizure foci in patients with medically intractable epilepsy. *Epilepsia*. 2013;54(2):341-50.

32. C Kesavadas and B Thomas. Clinical applications of functional MRI in epilepsy. *Indian J Radiol Imaging*. 2008;18(3):210-17.

33. JP Szaflarski, D Gloss, JR Binder et al. Practice guideline summary: Use of fMRI in the presurgical evaluation of patients with epilepsy: Report of the Guideline Development, Dissemination, and Implementation Subcommittee of the American Academy of Neurology. *Neurology*. 2017;88(4):395-402.

34. M Zijlmans, G Huiskamp, M Hersevoort et al. EEG-fMRI in the preoperative work-up for epilepsy surgery. *Brain*. 2007;130(pt. 9):2343-53.

6

How Do I Care for Patients in the Emergency Department and Inpatient Settings?

First-Time Seizure Review

First seizure management is covered comprehensively in Chapter 1. Still, we provide a brief synopsis of that chapter here, including expedited history, antiseizure medicine (ASM) decision making, and ancillary work-up. As for any acute medical situation, the first step in a first seizure is ensuring the seizure has ended and the patient is not in status epilepticus.

Key Points for Obtaining a History of a First-Time Seizure

The first goal of obtaining clinical details is to *determine if the event is indeed an epileptic seizure* or instead a nonepileptic paroxysmal event, whether organic or functional. Syncope, transient ischemic attack, migraine, and movement disorders comprise the main differential for seizures. Thus, clinical history should focus on ruling these out.

The most important component of first-time seizure evaluation is the clinical history. It is important to obtain information about the event *from both a witness and the patient.*

The witness can provide objective information, particularly crucial if there is loss of awareness. Ask the witness about the patient's acute

- Appearance (pallor versus cyanosis, other autonomic signs)
- Muscle tone
- Eye position
- Presence of abnormal movements (single versus intermittent versus repetitive, rhythmic versus arrhythmic, start/stop quality, symmetric versus asymmetric, violent, mouth/hand automatisms)
- Ictal cry
- Presence of stertorous breathing
- Blood or mouth foaming
- Bowel/urinary incontinence
- Responsiveness during the event
- Changes in behavior
- Presence of focal signs
- Length of time to return to cognitive baseline.

The patient will be able to provide information about additional *subjective symptoms* that are not visible to the witness' eyes. While the patient's entire recollection of the episode is important, the very first symptom is critical. The presence of auras or other prodromal symptoms can be diagnostic for both seizures and nonepileptic diagnoses. An easy question to use here is, "What was the first thing you noticed as this started happening to you?"

A specific diagnosis for seizure and other seizure mimics depends not only on the sign/symptoms, but also the *evolution* in which the symptoms develop over the duration of the event. Other essential features include:

- Initial activity at that time of the event (i.e., sitting/standing, sleeping, etc.)
- Injuries (tongue biting, shoulder dislocations, fractures, bruises, etc.) that may have resulted as a consequence of the event. Shoulder dislocations and lateral tongue biting (as opposed to biting the tip of the tongue) are highly suggestive of convulsive seizure. Physical examination is critical here to identify focal neurological signs and cutaneous stigmata.

Once you have established a seizure diagnosis, next ascertain the possibility of a *provoked or acute symptomatic* etiology. Assess for common causes like alcohol withdrawal, use of drugs or medications that lower the seizure threshold, possible metabolic derangements, central nervous system (CNS) infection, head injury, stroke, and so on. This is important, as long-term ASM treatment is unlikely necessary in a provoked situation or acute symptomatic seizures. Alternatively, key features of a potential epilepsy diagnosis include personal risk factors for epilepsy (i.e., significant remote head trauma), family history of epilepsy, or other neurological diagnoses.

Once you have determined a "first" seizure as your diagnosis, *confirm it is indeed a first-time seizure.* Multiple different seizure types including dyscognitive/absence seizures, myoclonic seizures, episodic auras, or nocturnal seizures often are unrecognized before the patient presents to you with a bilateral tonic clonic seizure. If these seizures have occurred, you no longer have a first seizure, so the decision to start an ASM is more straightforward.

Does the Patient Need an ASM?

Simply put, ASMs should only be started if the patient has epilepsy. Antiseizure medicines are initiated when the diagnostic criteria for epilepsy is fulfilled [1]. The following items should be considered:

- The diagnosis of an epileptic syndrome confers an epilepsy diagnosis by definition. However, there are certain epileptic syndromes, particularly those corresponding to self-limited focal epilepsies of childhood, in which ASM treatment is not mandatory (and generally, not recommended). In that case, seizure frequency and impact of the seizures in the patient's quality of life may guide decision making.
- In cases in which the diagnosis of epilepsy is unclear but there is a threatening risk for the patient if another seizure occurs (i.e., a

generalized tonic clonic seizure in a patient receiving anticoagulant treatment), initiation of ASM may be considered on a case-by-case basis.

The ASM should be chosen by considering the patient's specific epilepsy or seizure type, comorbidities, and potential ASM side effects and drug interactions. If the epilepsy type is unclear, use broad-spectrum medications. Chapter 3 covers ASM choice and counseling in detail.

Role of Imaging

The role of imaging in the emergency setting is focused on ruling out intracranial pathology that requires immediate intervention. Computerized tomography (CT) is the imaging of choice in the emergency department due to its availability and rapidity in providing results.

On a nonemergent basis, a brain magnetic resonance image (MRI) with epilepsy protocol can more specifically evaluate for specific epilepsy etiologies. A brain MRI could be waived in patients fulfilling diagnostic criteria for an idiopathic generalized epilepsy syndrome in the absence of atypical features [2]. Neuroimaging is extensively discussed in Chapter 5.

Role of Electroencephalogram

Electroencephalogram (EEG) is helpful in determining the presence of abnormalities that may predispose the patient to epileptic seizures. The yield of the EEG is maximal if performed within 24 hours after the event, followed by a sleep-deprived EEG if needed [2]. Data from EEG can be used to inform ASM decisions. The types of EEGs, interpretation of reports, and representative EEG samples are found in Chapter 4.

Role of Labs

Basic blood work including complete blood count (CBC) and complete metabolic panel (CMP) should be performed. This assesses for potential causes of a provoked or acute symptomatic as well as other disorders resembling an epileptic seizure. Additional testing, such as lumbar puncture, urinary analysis, and so on, is indicated if there is clinical suspicion for an infectious process. Other testing should be performed based on clinical suspicion (dimer-D for pulmonary embolism, cardiac enzymes if chest pain, etc.). Drug screening can also be performed for additional consideration of a provoked seizure.

What Do I Do for Patients with Breakthrough Seizures with Known Epilepsy?

KEY HISTORY

Patients with established epilepsy may present to the emergency room due to breakthrough seizures. The goal of the assessment is to find out why a breakthrough seizure has occurred. The following are key questions you can assess to help in your decision making.

- Is the patient compliant with medications?
- What is the patient's baseline seizure frequency? When was their last seizure prior to the breakthrough? If the patient has drug-resistant epilepsy, there may be no identifiable cause of the breakthrough seizure.
- Are these the patient's typical seizures? If not, how are they different?
- Have there been any recent changes to the patient's ASM regimen, whether initiation, discontinuation, switching to generic, or other formulation change?

- Have there been any recent changes (initiation or discontinuation) in non-ASMs? Specifically ask about antibiotics, oral contraceptives, neuroleptics, antidepressants, and anxiolytics. Some of these medications can lower the seizure threshold. Table 8.1 provides a nonexhaustive list of these medications.
- Is there a current infection or illness? Ask for fever, sick contacts, cough, difficulty breathing, nausea/vomiting/diarrhea, tooth infections, urinary tract infection symptoms, and so on.
- Is the patient pregnant?
- Was there a lack of sleep recently?
- Are there new stressors?

Diagnostic Testing

The indications for different tests depend on the possible etiology of the breakthrough seizure. Lab work is regularly obtained. Complete blood count and CMP are usually performed in most patients to identify either potential systemic or metabolic derangements that may have contributed to lowering of the seizure threshold or signs of intercurrent infections. Drug testing is usually performed if there is suspicion for drug abuse. Antiseizure medicine levels are routinely performed for breakthrough seizures. Determining ASM concentrations in breakthrough seizures is indicated for [3]:

- Assessing compliance
- Determining potential alterations in steady-state ASM concentration due to changes in formulations
- Assessing potential alterations in pharmacokinetics (due to drug interactions, pregnancy, age-related factors, low protein state, etc.).

Neither neuroimaging nor EEG is usually indicated unless:

- The patient presents with new semiology
- The patient has a new focal neurological exam
- The patient does not return to baseline

- The patient is in status epilepticus
- There is concern for intracranial injury due to the seizure (i.e., the patient hit his head during the seizure), or a new intracranial process cannot be ruled out.

You may consider *other tests* if an infectious etiology is suspected:

- A chest x-ray and urinalysis are readily available in the emergency room and performed in many patients with good ASM compliance and without an evident infectious focus by anamnesis or physical exam.
- A lumbar puncture if fever without an identifiable infectious focus or if there is presence of meningeal signs or epidemiological context of risk.
- Additional specific tests should be performed depending on the clinical judgment according to the suspected etiology of seizure breakthrough.

Acute Management for a Breakthrough Seizure in Known Epilepsy

There are currently no guidelines regarding management of patients with breakthrough seizures. The goal is to ensure that the patient is clinically stable and to identify and address the potential triggers of the breakthrough.

As with any acute clinical scenario, the first step is to stabilize the patient. If actively seizing, assess ABC (airway, breathing, circulation). If there is concern for status epilepticus (seizure lasting longer than 5 minutes), lorazepam 4 mg intravenous (IV) should be administered. Chapter 7 addresses status epilepticus more comprehensively.

Lastly, we conclude this section with several typical scenarios for epilepsy patients.

(1) Breakthrough seizures in the context of noncompliance: There is no need for adjustments of the patient's baseline ASM dosing. Instead, first assess reasons of noncompliance. Next provide strategies to

ensure good compliance like a pill box, medication alarm, and so on. Antiseizure medicine levels may be considered to verify noncompliance, but are often not needed. Consider administering an extra dose or a loading dose. This can be (and often is) administered empirically. Although not required, if ASM levels are available, the following formula can be used: Loading dose = C × W × Vd, where C is the desired change in serum concentration (mg/L), W is the patient's weight (kg), and Vd is the estimated volume of distribution for the drug (L/kg).

(2) Breakthrough seizures in the context of recent ASM dose lowering: One should modify or resume prior ASM regimen. Antiseizure medicine levels are not typically needed.

(3) Breakthrough seizures in the context of pharmacokinetic changes (age-related changes, pregnancy, drug–drug interactions): Adjust home dose regimen with strong consideration of checking ASM levels. Consider replacing the medication responsible for the pharmacokinetic interaction if possible. If the patient is pregnant, obstetric evaluation to assess fetal well-being.

(4) Breakthrough seizures in the context of acute illness or metabolic derangement: Treat the underlying cause. Extra ASM(s) may be necessary during the acute illness. If seizure-free prior to the acute illness, it is reasonable to have a plan to return to the ASM dosing strategy prior to the acute illness. Antiseizure medicine levels are not often required.

(5) No apparent etiology for the breakthrough seizures after thorough work-up: Consider optimizing ASM regimen by increasing existing ASMs or adding a new ASM. Monitor closely in the upcoming weeks to assess clinical response. This scenario is common in the context of drug-resistant epilepsy. If a patient has previously failed more than two to three doses, consider reaching out to the patient's neurologist to discuss possible ASM adjustments in these challenging, but unfortunately common situation.

HOW DO I MANAGE PATIENTS IN THE PERIOPERATIVE PERIOD, RENAL FAILURE/ DIALYSIS, AND LIVER FAILURE?

Perioperative ASM Management

Patient's ASM regimen can be altered for multiple reasons during the perioperative period, including fasting, swallowing difficulties, postoperative vomiting, changes in absorption after gastrointestinal surgery, and so on [4]. There are currently no official guidelines on perioperative management of ASMs in patients with epilepsy. Therefore, the main goal is to avoid disruption of the home antiepileptic regimen during the perioperative period.

(1) In a case of elective surgery, the patient should be advised to take their habitual home ASMs until surgery with small sips of water. During the period that the oral route (PO) is not available, ASMs should be replaced by the equivalent IV form if available. The following parenteral ASMs are commercially available in the United States, with an equivalent oral dose listed [4].

- Phenobarbital: PO = IV
- Phenytoin: 100 mg phenytoin sodium PO = 90 mg phenytoin sodium IV
- Valproic acid: PO = IV
- Levetiracetam: PO = IV
- Brivaracetam: PO = IV
- Lacosamide: PO = IV
- Lorazepam: PO = IV.

(2) Although uncommonly administered rectally (PR), lamotrigine (60 mg PO = 100 mg PR) [4–6] and topiramate (PO = PR) [4, 7] can be administered rectally from oral capsules.

(3) For those ASMs in which there is no parenteral equivalent, consider administering the total daily dose in one dose before surgery.

(4) If PO intake of the typical ASM regimen is foreseen to be unavailable for >24 hours, consider a temporary switch to an ASM with available parenteral formulation. Once safe to reinitiate PO intake, consider administering a loading dose of the temporarily discontinued ASM. Antiseizure medicine levels may help in calculating the loading dose, although some ASM levels are not readily available [4].

ASM adjustment in renal and hepatic impairment is a common reason for consultation. Table 6.1 lists renal or hepatic considerations for each ASM.

Is Treatment Different for Acute Symptomatic Seizures and Provoked Seizures?

Short-term management of acute symptomatic seizures is different from unprovoked seizures [8]. Still, for both entities, long-term treatment is not indicated since enduring predisposition for seizures is no longer present – or more simply, the patient does not have epilepsy.

Confusingly, acute symptomatic seizures and provoked seizures are often used indistinguishably [9, 10]. More accurately, "acute symptomatic seizures" occur in concert with an acute CNS structural abnormality. In contrast, "provoked seizures" occur in the setting of an acute systemic derangement [11]. Although by definition, acute symptomatic and provoked seizures do not recur once the precipitating factor is corrected, a challenge of long-term prognostication is that acute CNS pathologies are associated with increased risk for later development of epilepsy [10].

Acute symptomatic seizures are seizures occurring within a week of an acute CNS injury. Examples of specific CNS injuries include stroke (ischemic or hemorrhagic), traumatic brain injury (which includes brain surgery), CNS infection, or first-presenting-symptom of multiple sclerosis relapse. Several considerations should be taken into account:

Table 6.1 Renal or hepatic considerations for each ASM

Drug	Renal impairment	Hepatic impairment
Phenobarbital	HD: Usual dose q12–16h Supplement with 50% usual dose after HD if the next maintenance dose is not due right after it PD: 50% usual dose q12–16h; consider supplement	Decrease dose, amount not defined
Phenytoin	Avoid oral load Monitor using the unbound fraction HD/PD: Avoid oral load No supplement dose required Monitor using the unbound fraction	Avoid oral load Monitor using unbound fraction
Carbamazepine	No adjustment required HD/PD: No adjustment required	Not defined. Caution advised
Oxcarbazepine	CrCl<30: Initiate at 150 mg q12h; increase slowly to achieve desired clinical response HD/PD: No supplement dose required	Mild to moderate: No adjustment Severe: Not defined
Eslicarbazepine	CrCl<50: Start at 200 mg q24h After 2 weeks, increase to 400 mg q24h (recommended maintenance dose) Max. maintenance dose: 600 mg q24h HD/PD: Not defined	Mild to moderate: No adjustment Severe: Not defined. Avoid eslicarbazepine

Drug	Renal adjustment	Hepatic adjustment
Lamotrigine	Caution advised HD: Consider supplementing dose	Mild: No adjustment Moderate or severe without ascites: Reduce all doses by 25% Severe impairment with ascites: Reduce dose by 50%
Lacosamide	CrCl>30: No adjustment CrCl<30: Max. 300 mg/day, in two doses HD: Max. 300 mg/day and supplement of 50% the usual dose after HD session PD: Not defined	Mild to moderate: Max. 300 mg/day Severe: Avoid lacosamide
Valproic acid	No adjustment HD/PD: No adjustment or supplement dose required. Monitor using unbound fraction	Valproic acid is contraindicated in hepatic disorders or hepatic dysfunction
Levetiracetam	CrCl 50–80: 500–1,000 mg q12h CrCl 30–50: 250–750 mg q12h CrCl<30: 250–500 mg q12h HD/PD: 500–1,000 mg q24h and 250–500 mg supplemental dose after HD session	No adjustment

Table 6.1 (cont.)

Drug	Renal impairment	Hepatic impairment
Brivaracetam	No adjustment No data in ESRD HD/PD: Not defined	**Adults (≥16 years) or pediatric patients ≥50 kg** • Max. initial dose: 25 mg q12h • Max. maintenance dose: 75 mg q12h **Pediatric patients 20–50 kg** • Max. initial dose: 0.5 mg/kg q12h • Max. maintenance dose: 1.5 mg/kg q12h **Pediatric patients 11–20 kg** • Max. initial dose: 0.5 mg/kg q12h • Max. maintenance dose: 2 mg/kg q12h **Pediatric patients <11 kg** • Max. initial dose: 0.75 mg/kg q12h • Max. maintenance dose: 2.25 mg/kg q12h
Topiramate	CrCl<70: Reduce usual dose by 50% HD: Supplement 50% of daily dose after each session	Not defined. Caution advised
Zonisamide	Not defined CrCl<20: Gradually titrate from initial low dose HD: Supplement 200–400 mg after each session	Not defined

Drug		
PER	Mild RI: No adjustment	Mild: Start 2 mg q24h and increase by 2 mg q24h no more often than q2wk. Max. dose 6 mg q24h
	Moderate RI: Close monitoring, consider slower titration	Moderate: Start 2 mg q24h and increase by 2 mg q24h no more often than q2wk. Max. dose 4 mg q24h
	Severe RI: Avoid	Severe: Avoid
	HD/PD: Avoid	
Clobazam	Mild and moderate: No adjustment	Mild to moderate: Starting dose 5 mg q24h; titrate decreasing by 50% the recommended dose
	Severe: Not defined	Severe: Not defined
Pregabalin	CrCl 30–60: 75–300 mg/day, in two or three doses	No adjustment
	CrCl 15–30: 25–150 mg/day, in one or two doses	
	CrCl<15: 25–75 mg/day, in one dose	
	HD: Supplementary dose needed according to habitual dose:	
	• If 25 mg q24h ≥ supplement dose of 25 or 50 mg	
	• If 25–50 mg q24h ≥ supplement dose of 50 or 75 mg	
	• If 50–75 mg q24h ≥ supplement dose of 75–100 mg	
	• If 75 mg q24h ≥ supplement dose of 100–150 mg	

Table 6.1 (cont.)

Drug	Renal impairment	Hepatic impairment
Gabapentin	CrCl 30–59: 400–1400 mg/day, in two doses CrCl 15–29: 200–700 mg/day, in two doses CrCl<15: 100–300 mg/day in one dose. Caution HD: Supplementary dose 125–350 mg	Not adjustment
Vigabatrin	Pediatric patients 10 years and older, and adult patients CrCl>50–80: Decrease by 25% CrCl>30–50: Decrease by 50% CrCl>10–30: Decrease by 75% CrCl<11: Not defined HD/PD: Not defined	Not defined
Cannabidiol	No adjustment HD/PD: Not defined	Mild: • Starting dose: 2.5 mg/kg q12h • Maintenance dose: 5 mg/kg q12h • Max. recommended dose: 10 mg/kg q12 h Moderate: • Starting dose: 1.25 mg/kg q12h • Maintenance dose: 2.5 mg/kg q12h • Max. recommended dose: 5 mg/kg q12h

Rufinamide	No adjustment	Severe: • Starting dose: 0.5 mg/kg q12h • Maintenance dose: 1 mg/kg q12h • Max. recommended dose: 2 mg/kg q12h Mild and moderate: Caution Severe: Avoid rufinamide
	HD: No adjustment. Supplement of 30% the usual dose after session PD: Not defined	
Felbamate	Reduce habitual dose by 50% HD/PD: No data	Felbamate is contraindicated

CrCl: creatinine clearance (expressed in ml/min); ESRD: end-stage renal disease; HD: hemodialysis; PD: peritoneal dialysis; PER: perampanel; q12h: every 12 hours; q24h: every 24 hours; q2wk: every 2 weeks; RI: renal impairment

- For CNS infections, acute symptomatic seizures can extend beyond the 7-day period with persistence of active infection. Specific criteria are used for malaria, neurocysticercosis, brain abscess, and HIV [12].
- Seizures in the presence of an arteriovenous malformation are considered acute symptomatic only during acute hemorrhage. Arteriovenous malformations are common causes of epilepsy.

Prophylactic ASMs do not decrease the incidence of developing epilepsy, but can be used in the immediate management of acute symptomatic seizures. Antiseizure medicine should be chosen by considering the patient's comorbidities, drug interactions, and side effects, as described in Chapter 3. For example, in a case of intracranial hemorrhage, valproic acid should be avoided due to possible thrombocytopenia and platelet dysfunction.

A common challenge of ASM management for acute symptomatic seizures is when to stop treatment. No guidelines address ASM taper after acute symptomatic seizures [13]. In clinical practice, if seizures do not recur after 3–6 months and extended EEG does not show epileptiform abnormalities, ASMs are often discontinued.

Provoked seizures are those that occur in the setting of a severe, acute (within 24 hours) metabolic derangement, illicit drugs use, alcohol intoxication or withdrawal, benzodiazepine/barbiturate withdrawal, or use of medications that are known to lower the seizure threshold [11]. The goal in the emergency department is to correct such disturbances and identify and treat the underlying cause. Seizures are generalized tonic clonic without any focal features per history or neurological exam. However, focal seizures have been documented in the setting of nonketotic hyperglycemia [14, 15].

The International League Against Epilepsy has established the cut-off values for several metabolic disturbances in order to be considered as the provoking factors for seizures [9]:

- Serum glucose <36 mg/dL or >450 mg/dL associated with ketoacidosis
- Serum sodium <115 mg/dL

- Serum calcium <5 mg/dL
- Serum magnesium <0.8 mg/dL
- Urea nitrogen >100 mg/dL
- Creatinine >10 mg/dL.

The following sections list specific common etiologies of provoked seizures.

PROVOKED SEIZURES RELATED TO ALCOHOL AND ILLICIT DRUGS

Both alcohol withdrawal and alcohol abuse can lead to an epileptic seizure.

- Alcohol withdrawal: Consider alcohol withdrawal seizures if there is a personal history of chronic alcohol abuse, with or without a recent reduction in consumption, and if there are accompanying symptoms of withdrawal, such as tremors, diaphoresis, or tachycardia.
  - Seizure must occur within 7–48 hours of the last drink [9].
  - Seizure should occur with alcohol blood levels close to 0.
  - Seizure should be a generalized tonic clonic seizure.
  - Other etiologies for acute symptomatic seizures should be ruled out, particularly if focal symptoms or signs or status epilepticus.
- Alcohol abuse: Consider this possibility in a patient in which there is no history of chronic alcohol abuse but there is documented recent alcohol abuse, such as weekend binge alcohol consumption [9, 16].

  Alcohol withdrawal syndrome, of which alcohol withdrawal seizures is part, is a life-threatening situation and should be treated as such:

- Benzodiazepines IV (diazepam or lorazepam) are the medication of choice to avoid seizure recurrence and other alcohol withdrawal symptoms.
- Thiamine IV should be administered in every patient to prevent Wernicke–Korsakov syndrome. Carbohydrate-containing fluids or

food should not be started without prior thiamine administration. Additional nutritional support is recommended.

- Close clinical monitoring is recommended. Consider transferring to ICU.
- Any accompanying metabolic imbalance should be corrected.
- Support treatment according to clinical judgment.
- Status epilepticus management (covered in Chapter 7) is no different for this clinical entity.

Cocaine and amphetamines have been reported to produce epileptic seizures within hours of use. Given the risk of intracranial hemorrhage or vasospasm, neuroimaging should be considered. Treatment of seizures is supportive with more direct management of other intracranial complications as required.

BENZODIAZEPINE AND BARBITURATE WITHDRAWAL

Similar to alcohol withdrawal seizures, abrupt cessation of sedatives such as benzodiazepines, barbiturates, and zolpidem can produce withdrawal seizures [16]. Seizures have also been reported with the use of flumazenil in patients with benzodiazepine withdrawal symptoms or that have been recently treated with benzodiazepines [17].

Treatment is benzodiazepines and supportive. Once the patient is stabilized, if a benzodiazepine use disorder is suspected, consider referral to psychiatry for an adequate benzodiazepine tapering.

IATROGENIC MEDICATION–INDUCED PROVOKED SEIZURES

Commonly used medications in clinical practice are known to lower the seizure threshold. Treatment of iatrogenically induced seizures is cessation of the precipitating agent. In case of status epilepticus,

Table 6.2 List of commonly used drugs that may lower seizure threshold

Antimicrobials	Penicillins
	Cephalosporins (particularly cefepime)
	Carbapenems (particularly imipenem)
	Fluoroquinolones
	Isoniazid
	Mefloquine and chloroquine
Analgesics	Tramadol
Antipsychotics	Clozapine
	Other antipsychotics modestly lower risk
	Note this is not a contraindication to use in patients with epilepsy
Antidepressants	Bupropion
	Overdose of the tricyclic class

treatment should not differ from other etiologies. See Table 6.2 for a list of commonly used drugs that may lower seizure threshold [18].

Of note, *cefepime-induced encephalopathy* is increasingly encountered in the ICU setting. Cefepime encephalopathy can progress to seizures and status epilepticus (characteristically nonconvulsive or myoclonic status epilepticus). It typically starts 2–6 days after cefepime initiation and renal impairment is a common risk factor. Cefepime-induced encephalopathy may require hemodialysis [19]. Electroencephalogram shows generalized periodic discharges, at times with triphasic morphology [19, 20]. These are sometimes difficult to differentiate from a nonconvulsive status epilepticus and Salzburg criteria should be utilized to establish the diagnosis [21].

Isoniazid-induced seizures occur due to inhibition of pyridoxine phosphokinase, which decreases pyridoxal-5-phosphate, an essential cofactor for the synthesis of GABA. Isoniazid-induced seizures are responsive to pyridoxine and benzodiazepines.

How Do I Manage Patients Admitted to the Epilepsy Monitoring Unit

Patients admitted to the epilepsy monitoring unit (EMU) are one of the select populations of asymptomatic patients admitted for the express intent of causing their clinical symptoms. This section discusses testing during paroxysmal events, titrating ASMs, and patient safety during the admission.

Testing/Treating a Patient during a Paroxysmal Event

An EMU provides a unique setting for electroclinical characterization of a patient's events and is the gold standard for epilepsy and nonepileptic event classification. Given the time sacrifice a patient makes to be in the EMU, every effort should be made to obtain the most information possible from the events recorded in the EMU. Thus, we provide guidance on steps to be taken before a seizure occurs, the evaluation during a seizure, and continued evaluation after the seizure concludes [22].

- Before the seizure and at seizure onset
  - All patients should have IV access placed on admission
  - Patient beds should have extra padding to help protect the patient during a seizure
  - Emergency IV epilepsy medications (i.e., benzodiazepines) should be immediately available
  - Ensure the camera is focused on the patient
  - Have supplies to treat a convulsive seizure including oxygen and suction made ready before the seizure
  - Physicians capable of managing epilepsy emergencies should be available in house 24 hours a day.
- At seizure onset and during the seizure
  - As the seizure begins, the lights should be turned on and the patient uncovered while respecting patient privacy
  - Greet the patient by their name, which helps immediately assess for responsiveness. If the patient does not respond, try touching their arm

- Staff should describe the patient's aspect: color, sweatiness, piloerection, sialorrhea, subtle movements, or eye deviation
- As details may not be visualized on camera, any of these changes should be verbalized aloud
- If the patient is aware, try to obtain thorough description of the aura that they are feeling, if any. This should include laterality and localization of symptoms
- Provide a key phrase (i.e., green horse) that can be later used to test memory
- Test for comprehension by asking the patient to complete movements. It is vital not to perform the movement, as patients can mime the response without true comprehension
- Ask patients to speak simple items like their names and more complicated items like recent current events
- Most importantly, even if they cannot fully respond to your testing/commands, continue to test the patient to ascertain any fluctuation in cognitive status.

- If there is a convulsive phase of the seizure
  - The patient should be rolled on to their side, taking care to make sure limbs are not being restrained by a person or objects (i.e., the bed)
  - Oxygen should be applied, preferentially via a face mask delivery if available
  - While suction may be used to remove saliva, nothing should be placed in the patient's mouth
  - For seizures lasting longer than 4 minutes, an IV benzodiazepine should be administered according to local practice
  - While rarely occurring, supplies for cardiopulmonary resuscitation should be immediately available.

- After the seizure
  - Assess for recollection of the event: "What just happened?" "Did you have a seizure?" "What do you remember?" "Do you remember the word/color that I asked you to remember?"

- Test for language and orientation as discussed earlier during the ictal period
- Ask the patient to describe the seizure. In case of a visual aura, ask the patient to draw it
- Continue to frequently assess the patient until back at their baseline
- Confirm with the patient or caregivers that the event captured was the patient's habitual events.

ASM Titration during an EMU Admission

To properly characterize patients' epilepsy, a sufficient number of habitual seizures should be recorded during an EMU admission. The duration of the admission may be a limiting constraint for seizure recording. Thus, provoking measures such as photic stimulation, hyperventilation, sleep deprivation, and ASM tapering are commonly performed.

A common question for patients and physicians alike is how to titrate ASMs during an admission. A randomized controlled study compared rapid (30–50% daily ASM dose reduction) versus slow (15–30% daily ASM dose reduction) ASM tapering.

The study showed rapid tapering is associated with:

- Shorter monitoring duration
- Shorter time to first seizure
- A higher incidence of seizure clusters (>3 seizures in 4 hours).

No difference was seen in use of rescue medication or occurrence of secondary generalized seizures between rapid and slow tapering. There was no difference in the diagnostic yield, although this could be explained by the fact that monitoring was continued until enough seizures were recorded. Therefore, a rapid taper seems effective in shortening the admission duration without any major adverse effects [23].

Still, patient safety will always be the most important consideration during an EMU admission. A rational approach for ASM withdrawal has been outlined, considering the habitual seizure frequency and the home ASM regimen [24]:

- Consider no ASM withdrawal if the patient has two or more seizure per week or there is history of status epilepticus
- Consider preadmission withdrawal of long-acting ASMs (i.e., perampanel, zonisamide, etc.) if the criteria mentioned are not present
- Consider slow titration, if any, of clobazam, clonazepam, and phenobarbital as abrupt discontinuation can trigger withdrawal seizures
- Consider gradual tapering of ASMs with short half-lives (levetiracetam, brivaracetam, carbamazepine, oxcarbazepine, and lacosamide) to avoid a rapid drop in serum levels
- Consider abrupt cessation of intermediate half-life ASMs (ethosuximide, eslicarbazepine, lamotrigine, and topiramate).

Monitoring for the Patient's Safety

While observing the recommendations and appropriate clinical common sense, the nature of the EMU monitoring does place your patient at risk for clusters and prolonged seizures, status epilepticus, falls, and, infrequently, death [25].

To minimize this risk, it is critical to implement specific, standardized safety protocols. The following aspects should be considered [25]:

- *Preadmission assessment* determines plans for observation and safety by preemptively assessing injury risk and comorbid conditions that could be exacerbated because of seizures. The patient and relatives should be educated about the intended procedures during admission.
- All staff on an EMU should receive proper *training* in epilepsy and acute seizure management. This should include seizure recognition and reporting, clinical assessment during seizures, medication management, seizure first aid, and management of seizure emergencies.

- Continuous observation is required due to the unpredictable timing of seizures during an EMU admission. This is particularly imperative during intracranial EEG. Automated seizure detection can assist, but does not replace human monitoring. While family members, friends, or caregivers are often present, they also do not replace continuous professional observation. It should be performed with direct observation or closed-circuit camera. Monitoring staff should be specifically trained in the use of EEG telemetry and able to recognize EEG or behavioral changes indicative of possible seizures. Pulse oximetry and cardiac monitoring should be conducted with a minimum of single-lead EKG.

- *Daily assessment* should include changes in mental status and behavior, ongoing log of seizures and administered medication, including rescue seizure medication. The integrity of EEG electrodes and the quality of the EEG recording should be ensured. For intracranial patients, the integrity of the head wrap and presence of drainage or bleeding should also be evaluated.

- *Environment and activities* involve designing patient room and bathroom facilities to minimize the risk of injury. Staff should assist patients when using the restroom. Exercise equipment can be used with supervision. Higher safety restrictions may be needed in intracranial EEG patients to protect from displacing the electrodes.

- *Discharge planning* considers the time of the last seizure, generally allowing for a 24-hour seizure-free period prior to discharge or ensuring stability in the baseline seizure rate for that patient. The patient and relatives are instructed regarding acute rescue medications and when to call for help as well as when to contact their epileptologist for changes in seizures or behavior/mood (i.e., postictal psychosis). The patient and relatives should be informed about the ASM changes during admission and about the medication regimen that is indicated after discharge. Temporary safety precautions such as possible activity limitations and timing to resume normal activity should be directly addressed since ASMs were held. Lastly, follow-up appointments should be formally addressed.

Works Cited

1. RS Fisher, C Acevedo, A Arzimanoglou et al. ILAE official report: A practical clinical definition of epilepsy. *Epilepsia*. 2014;55(4):475-82.

2. MA King, MR Newton, GD Jackson et al. Epileptology of the first-seizure presentation: A clinical, electroencephalographic, and magnetic resonance imaging study of 300 consecutive patients. *Lancet*. 1998;352(9133):1007-11.

3. PN Patsalos, DJ Berry, BF Bourgeois et al. Antiepileptic drugs – Best practice guidelines for therapeutic drug monitoring: A position paper by the subcommission on therapeutic drug monitoring, ILAE Commission on Therapeutic Strategies. *Epilepsia*. 2008;49(7):1239-76.

4. WS Wichards, AF Schobben, and FS Leijten. Perioperative substitution of anti-epileptic drugs. *J Neurol*. 2013;260(11):2865-75.

5. AK Birnbaum, RL Kriel, RT Burkhardt, and RP Remmel. Rectal absorption of lamotrigine compressed tablets. *Epilepsia*. 2000;41(7):850-3.

6. AK Birnbaum, RL Kriel, Y Im, and RP Remmel. Relative bioavailability of lamotrigine chewable dispersible tablets administered rectally. *Pharmacotherapy*. 2001;21(2):158-62.

7. JM Conway, AK Birnbaum, RL Kriel, and JC Cloyd. Relative bioavailability of topiramate administered rectally. *Epilepsy Res*. 2003;54(2-3):91-6.

8. K Verhaert and RC Scott. Acute Symptomatic Epileptic Seizures. In: CP Panayiotopoulos, editor. *Atlas of Epilepsies*. London: Springer London; 2010. 69-78.

9. E Beghi, A Carpio, L Forsgren et al. Recommendation for a definition of acute symptomatic seizure. *Epilepsia*. 2010;51(4):671-5.

10. M Mauritz, LJ Hirsch, P Camfield et al. Acute symptomatic seizures: An educational, evidence-based review. *Epileptic Disord*. 2022;24(1):26-49.

11. E Wyllie, BE Gidal, HP Goodkin, L Jehi, and T Loddenkemper. *Wyllie's Treatment of Epilepsy: Principles and Practice*. Philadelphia: Wolters Kluwer; 2020.

12. DJ Thurman, E Beghi, CE Begley et al. Standards for epidemiologic studies and surveillance of epilepsy. *Epilepsia*. 2011;52(Suppl. 7):2-26.

13. V Punia, P Chandan, J Fesler, CR Newey, and S Hantus. Post-acute symptomatic seizure (PASS) clinic: A continuity of care model for patients impacted by continuous EEG monitoring. *Epilepsia Open*. 2020;5(2):255-62.

14. F Moien-Afshari and JF Tellez-Zenteno. Occipital seizures induced by hyperglycemia: A case report and review of literature. *Seizure*. 2009;18(5):382–5.

15. A Hennis, D Corbin, and H Fraser. Focal seizures and non-ketotic hyperglycaemia. *J Neurol Neurosurg Psychiatry*. 1992;55(3):195–7.

16. TA Nowacki and JD Jirsch. Evaluation of the first seizure patient: Key points in the history and physical examination. *Seizure*. 2017;49:54–63.

17. WH Spivey. Flumazenil and seizures: Analysis of 43 cases. *Clin Ther*. 1992;14(2):292–305.

18. AW Hitchings. Drugs that lower the seizure threshold. *Adverse Drug React Bull*. 2016(298):1151–4.

19. LE Payne, DJ Gagnon, RR Riker et al. Cefepime-induced neurotoxicity: A systematic review. *Crit Care*. 2017;21(1):276.

20. HT Li, CH Lee, T Wu et al. Clinical, electroencephalographic features and prognostic factors of cefepime-induced neurotoxicity: A retrospective study. *Neurocrit Care*. 2019;31(2):329–37.

21. M Leitinger, S Beniczky, A Rohracher et al. Salzburg Consensus Criteria for Non-convulsive Status Epilepticus: Approach to clinical application. *Epilepsy Behav*. 2015;49:158–63.

22. S Beniczky, M Neufeld, B Diehl et al. Testing patients during seizures: A European consensus procedure developed by a joint taskforce of the ILAE – Commission on European Affairs and the European Epilepsy Monitoring Unit Association. *Epilepsia*. 2016;57(9):1363–8.

23. S Kumar, B Ramanujam, PS Chandra et al. Randomized controlled study comparing the efficacy of rapid and slow withdrawal of antiepileptic drugs during long-term video-EEG monitoring. *Epilepsia*. 2018;59(2):460–7.

24. J Kirby, VM Leach, A Brockington et al. Drug withdrawal in the epilepsy monitoring unit: The Patsalos table. *Seizure*. 2020;75:75–81.

25. PO Shafer, JM Buelow, K Noe et al. A consensus-based approach to patient safety in epilepsy monitoring units: Recommendations for preferred practices. *Epilepsy Behav*. 2012;25(3):449–56.

7

How Do I Manage Epilepsy Emergencies Like Status Epilepticus?

Definition of Status Epilepticus

Status epilepticus (SE) is a condition resulting from an abnormally long seizure or cluster without return to baseline neurological status. Status epilepticus is highly considered for a seizure lasting longer than 5 minutes, as seizure are unlikely to stop without treatment if longer than 5 minutes [1].

The time to irreversible neurological injury varies by SE type. For convulsive SE (CSE), the potential for long-term neuronal damage occurs after 30 minutes [1]. For focal SE with impaired awareness, irreversible neuronal damage can occur after 60 minutes [1]. The time range for irreversible neuronal injury with absence SE is not known. While data is limited for other types of nonconvulsive SE (NCSE), prompt treatment is recommended.

Clinical Features of CSE

Recognizing CSE is often not difficult and starts by recognizing the seizure semiology discussed in previous chapters. Limb movements should be rhythmic, synchronous, and not suppressible. The patient will be unconscious and most of the time the eyes will be open. Other clinical features include oral trauma, and either bowel or bladder incontinence.

Conversely, features indicating a nonepileptic event (so-called nonepileptic SE) include the opposite; namely, nonrhythmic or nonsynchronous movements, suppressible movements, maintained awareness, or the eyes being closed.

Nonconvulsive SE can be more difficult to recognize and is discussed in later sections of this chapter.

Treatment of SE

Early treatment is vital as longer duration of SE leads to: increased resistance to pharmacologic treatment, notably benzodiazepines [2], and increased mortality [3, 4].

STEP 1 – SEIZURE: 0–5 MINUTES

- Most seizures are self-limiting and stop within 2–3 minutes [5, 6]
- Place patient on their side if possible, free of obstacles, and prevent falls
- Time the seizure
- ABCs
  - Maintain airway
  - Administer oxygen with face mask
  - Start an IV
- Check blood glucose and consider thiamine up to 500 mg IV followed by or concurrent with 50 mL of D 50% [7, 8].

STEP 2 – EARLY SE: 5–10 MINUTES

- The first treatment is unequivocally an adequate dosing of a benzodiazepine. The biggest mistake here is underdosing [9]. Most adults can receive the following doses, with pediatric doses being weight based [7].

- Lorazepam 4 mg IV (0.1 mg/kg/dose with max. of 4 mg/dose, can repeat once if needed)
- Midazolam 10 mg IM if no IV access (10 mg if over 40 kg, 5 mg if 13–40 kg, do not repeat)
- Alternatives include: IV or rectal diazepam; intranasal or buccal midazolam.
- Studies have shown no difference in the need for intubation with benzodiazepines versus placebo in CSE, with one study showing a trend toward treatment with a benzodiazepine being protective against the need for intubation [10, 11].

STEP 3 – ESTABLISHED SE: 10–30 MINUTES

- If your patient continues to seize after appropriate benzodiazepine dosing; one of fosphenytoin, valproate, or levetiracetam can be used as each has been proven equally as efficacious [12]. It is ideal to avoid phenytoin due to the risk of chemical burn with IV infiltration [13].
  - IV fosphenytoin (20 mg/kg with a max. dose of 1,500 mg)
  - IV valproate (40 mg/kg with a max. dose of 3,000 mg)
  - IV levetiracetam (60 mg/kg with a max. dose of 4,500 mg).

STEP 4 – REFRACTORY SE: 30 MINUTES–24 HOURS

- Initiate video electroencephalogram (EEG) if available
- Intubate patient and admit to ICU if not already performed
- Third treatment – IV anesthetic [14]
  - IV propofol
  - IV midazolam
  - IV pentobarbital
- Treat the underlying etiology – identification of etiology is discussed later.

STEP 5 – SUPERREFRACTORY SE: BEYOND 24 HOURS AND FAILURE OF IV ANESTHETIC

- A comprehensive review is beyond the scope of this epilepsy manual. Still, in brief, superrefractory SE occurs in 20% of refractory SE patients [15]
- Superrefractory SE is best managed in conjunction with a neurointensivist and epilepsy specialist
  - Multiple treatment strategies have been considered for this cohort, including but not limited to ketamine [16], epilepsy surgery [17], ketogenic diet [18], and hypothermia [19].

Focal Motor SE

Focal motor SE refers to the prolonged, stereotyped, repetitive unilateral clonic activity of the face/arm/leg together or in isolation [20]. There can be fluctuation as the seizures briefly stop in between and crucially can persist in sleep [20]. Focal motor SE must be distinguished from potential mimics such as tremor or myoclonus to prevent unnecessary treatments [20].

Data are limited on the optimum time to treat and the consequences of prolonged focal motor SE. Sixty minutes has been suggested as the time at which to define and more aggressively treat [21]. However, treatment should be initiated as early as the SE is recognized. Because focal motor SE originates from discrete brain lesions, early brain imaging is a mainstay to determine an etiology that may be intervened upon. An EEG can be negative in up to 20% of cases [22].

Nonconvulsive SE

Nonconvulsive SE (NCSE) refers to prolonged seizure(s) that have no major motor semiology [23]. Nonconvulsive SE represents a varied spectrum of clinical and electrographic findings. Broadly these can be separated into four main categories of: focal with retained awareness (not including focal motor); focal with impaired awareness; absence; and SE in coma [23].

FOCAL WITH RETAINED AWARENESS

Clinical features can include any prolonged or repetitive aura, change in behavior, aphasia, eye deviation or nystagmus, simple unilateral visual hallucinations, or other focal neurologic symptoms [20]. An EEG can be without ictal correlate [22]. Suspicion should be highest in a patient with known focal epilepsy and repetitive manifestations of their typical seizure semiology.

FOCAL WITH IMPAIRED AWARENESS

Clinical features can include any of those seen with focal with retained awareness though with the obvious addition of loss of awareness. There may be subtle eye movements, unilateral motor involvement, automatisms, perseveration, or confusion [20]. An EEG is much more sensitive and likely to be diagnostic in focal SE with impaired awareness [24].

ABSENCE

Clinical features can be mild confusion to overt behavioral changes. Eyelid myoclonus can be present [20]. An EEG shows generalized ~3 Hz spike and wave. Suspicion should be highest in a patient with a known history of generalized epilepsy.

NCSE IN COMA

Nonconvulsive SE in coma is a diagnosis that requires both clinical and electrographic abnormalities. Coma can be the only clinical manifestation in 50–90% of cases [25–27]. The most common subtle signs are facial twitching and/or eye deviation [25, 28]. Due to the minimal or lack of clinical features, an EEG is required for diagnosis. Electroencephalogy terminology and criteria known as the Salzburg criteria is used to guide such a diagnosis [29]. Nonconvulsive SE in comatose patients is most common in patients who had witnessed seizure prior to coma [28, 30, 31]. Suspicion should also be high in patients with a history of epilepsy or neurological insult (e.g., intracranial tumor, meningitis/encephalitis, and remote or recent brain injury) [25, 28].

Etiology

As noted previously, determining the SE etiology is vital in guiding treatment. The underlying cause should be sought throughout the treatment process. There are many potential causes of SE, which include [14, 32]:

- Epilepsy specific causes: preexisting epilepsy with breakthrough seizure or antiseizure medicine (ASM) noncompliance, which is the most common cause of SE [33, 34]
- Vascular: hemorrhagic>ischemic stroke, cerebral venous sinus thrombosis, hypoxia, or posterior reversible encephalopathy syndrome (PRES)
- Infection: encephalitis, meningitis, abscess, or sepsis
- Traumatic: head trauma with or without hemorrhage
- Autoimmune: autoimmune encephalitis (anti-NMDA, anti-VGKC, etc.) or paraneoplastic
- Metabolic: hypoglycemia, renal failure, drug toxicity, or drug withdrawal (benzodiazepine, alcohol, barbiturate)
- Neoplastic: primary and metastatic central nervous system tumors.

It should be noted that any acute or chronic damage to the cortex can make it more likely to have a seizure and thus could present as SE.

Postcardiac Arrest

Status epilepticus after cardiac arrest is very common, seen in up to 30% of patients [35, 36]. Status epilepticus in this setting can present with convulsions, however most often it takes the form of NCSE or myoclonic SE [36]. Generally, the onset of electrographic SE is between ~12 and ~48 hours after cardiac arrest, though it can occur outside of this time period [35]. Treatment does not differ from that of other types of SE. Both NCSE and myoclonic SE have been shown to indicate a poor prognosis after cardiac arrest [36–40].

The 2020 American Heart Association guidelines recommend prompt EEG for detection of seizures in patients who are comatose after resuscitation [41]. An EEG is also often used as a prognostic tool regardless of SE. Multiple studies have shown that lack of EEG reactivity or burst suppression after rewarming are poor prognostic indicators for neurological recovery with specificity near or at 100% in multiple studies [39, 42–44].

Works Cited

1. E Trinka, H Cock, D Hesdorffer et al. A definition and classification of status epilepticus: Report of the ILAE Task Force on Classification of Status Epilepticus. *Epilepsia*. 2015;56(10):1515–23.

2. J Kapur and RL Macdonald. Rapid seizure-induced reduction of benzodiazepine and Zn^{2+} sensitivity of hippocampal dentate granule cell GABAA receptors. *J Neurosci.* 1997;17(19):7532–40.

3. I Sánchez Fernández, HP Goodkin, and RC Scott. Pathophysiology of convulsive status epilepticus. *Seizure*. 2019;68:16–21.

4. RJ Lv, Q Wang, T Cui, F Zhu, and XQ Shao. Status epilepticus-related etiology, incidence and mortality: A meta-analysis. *Epilepsy Res*. 2017;136:12–17.

5. S Jenssen, EJ Gracely, and MR Sperling. How long do most seizures last? A systematic comparison of seizures recorded in the epilepsy monitoring unit. *Epilepsia*. 2006;47(9):1499–503.

6. WH Theodore, RJ Porter, P Albert et al. The secondarily generalized tonic-clonic seizure: A videotape analysis. *Neurology*. 1994;44(8):1403–7.

7. T Glauser, S Shinnar, D Gloss et al. Evidence-based guideline: Treatment of convulsive status epilepticus in children and adults: Report of the Guideline Committee of the American Epilepsy Society. *Epilepsy Curr*. 2016;16(1):48–61.

8. JP Betjemann and DH Lowenstein. Status epilepticus in adults. *Lancet Neurol*. 2015;14(6):615–24.

9. AG Sathe, E Underwood, LD Coles et al. Patterns of benzodiazepine underdosing in the Established Status Epilepticus Treatment Trial. *Epilepsia*. 2021;62(3):795–806.

10. BK Alldredge, DB Wall, and DM Ferriero. Effect of prehospital treatment on the outcome of status epilepticus in children. *Pediatr Neurol*. 1995;12(3):213–16.

11. BK Alldredge, AM Gelb, SM Isaacs et al. A comparison of lorazepam, diazepam, and placebo for the treatment of out-of-hospital status epilepticus. *N Engl J Med*. 2001;345(9):631–7.

12. J Kapur, J Elm, JM Chamberlain et al. Randomized Trial of Three Anticonvulsant Medications for Status Epilepticus. *N Engl J Med*. 2019;381(22):2103–13.

13. LA Garbovsky, BC Drumheller, and J Perrone. Purple glove syndrome after phenytoin or fosphenytoin administration: Review of reported cases and recommendations for prevention. *J Med Toxicol*. 2015;11(4):445–59.

14. GM Brophy, R Bell, J Claassen et al. Guidelines for the evaluation and management of status epilepticus. *Neurocrit Care*. 2012;17(1):3–23.

15. AM Kantanen, M Reinikainen, I Parviainen et al. Incidence and mortality of super-refractory status epilepticus in adults. *Epilepsy Behav*. 2015;49:131–4.

16. A Alkhachroum, CA Der-Nigoghossian, E Mathews et al. Ketamine to treat super-refractory status epilepticus. *Neurology*. 2020;95(16):e2286–94.

17. SD Lhatoo and AV Alexopoulos. The surgical treatment of status epilepticus. *Epilepsia*. 2007;48(Suppl. 8):61–5.

18. MC Cervenka, S Hocker, M Koenig et al. Phase I/II multicenter ketogenic diet study for adult superrefractory status epilepticus. *Neurology*. 2017;88(10):938–43.

19. JJ Corry, R Dhar, T Murphy, and MN Diringer. Hypothermia for refractory status epilepticus. *Neurocrit Care*. 2008;9(2):189–97.

20. MO Kinney, JJ Craig, and PW Kaplan. Non-convulsive status epilepticus: Mimics and chameleons. *Pract Neurol*. 2018;18(4):291–305.

21. R Mameniškienė and P Wolf. Epilepsia partialis continua: A review. *Seizure*. 2017;44:74–80.

22. R Mameniskiene, T Bast, C Bentes et al. Clinical course and variability of non-Rasmussen, nonstroke motor and sensory epilepsia partialis continua: A European survey and analysis of 65 cases. *Epilepsia*. 2011;52(6):1168–76.

23. H Meierkord and M Holtkamp. Non-convulsive status epilepticus in adults: Clinical forms and treatment. *Lancet Neurol.* 2007;6(4):329–39.

24. MJ Casale, LV Marcuse, JJ Young et al. The sensitivity of scalp EEG at detecting seizures: A simultaneous scalp and stereo EEG study. *J Clin Neurophysiol.* 2020;39(1):78–84.

25. AM Husain, GJ Horn, and MP Jacobson. Non-convulsive status epilepticus: Usefulness of clinical features in selecting patients for urgent EEG. *J Neurol Neurosurg Psychiatry.* 2003;74(2):189–91.

26. J Claassen, SA Mayer, RG Kowalski, RG Emerson, and LJ Hirsch. Detection of electrographic seizures with continuous EEG monitoring in critically ill patients. *Neurology.* 2004;62(10):1743–8.

27. JD Pandian, GD Cascino, EL So, E Manno, and JR Fulgham. Digital video-electroencephalographic monitoring in the neurological-neurosurgical intensive care unit: Clinical features and outcome. *Arch Neurol.* 2004;61(7):1090–4.

28. I Laccheo, H Sonmezturk, AB Bhatt et al. Non-convulsive status epilepticus and non-convulsive seizures in neurological ICU patients. *Neurocrit Care.* 2015;22(2):202–11.

29. S Beniczky, LJ Hirsch, PW Kaplan et al. Unified EEG terminology and criteria for nonconvulsive status epilepticus. *Epilepsia.* 2013;54(Suppl. 6):28–9.

30. P Kurtz, N Gaspard, AS Wahl et al. Continuous electroencephalography in a surgical intensive care unit. *Intensive Care Med.* 2014;40(2):228–34.

31. EJ Gilmore, N Gaspard, HA Choi et al. Acute brain failure in severe sepsis: A prospective study in the medical intensive care unit utilizing continuous EEG monitoring. *Intensive Care Med.* 2015;41(4):686–94.

32. E Trinka, J Höfler, and A Zerbs. Causes of status epilepticus. *Epilepsia.* 2012;53(Suppl. 4):127–38.

33. RJ DeLorenzo, WA Hauser, AR Towne et al. A prospective, population-based epidemiologic study of status epilepticus in Richmond, Virginia. *Neurology.* 1996;46(4):1029–35.

34. B Ozdilek, I Midi, K Agan, and CA Bingol. Episodes of status epilepticus in young adults: Etiologic factors, subtypes, and outcomes. *Epilepsy Behav.* 2013;27(2):351–4.

35. S Backman, E Westhall, I Dragancea et al. Electroencephalographic characteristics of status epilepticus after cardiac arrest. *Clin Neurophysiol.* 2017;128(4):681–8.

36. JC Rittenberger, A Popescu, RP Brenner, FX Guyette, and CW Callaway. Frequency and timing of nonconvulsive status epilepticus in comatose post-cardiac arrest subjects treated with hypothermia. *Neurocrit Care.* 2012;16(1):114–22.

37. MB Kelley, JA Wantuck, K Burns, and JA McPherson. The prevalence and prognostic value of myoclonus and status epilepticus prior to or following therapeutic hypothermia in patients after cardiac arrest. *J Am Coll Cardiol.* 2010;55(Suppl. 10):A111.E1037.

38. S Legriel, J Hilly-Ginoux, M Resche-Rigon et al. Prognostic value of electrographic postanoxic status epilepticus in comatose cardiac-arrest survivors in the therapeutic hypothermia era. *Resuscitation*. 2013;84(3):343–50.

39. A Sivaraju, EJ Gilmore, CR Wira et al. Prognostication of post-cardiac arrest coma: Early clinical and electroencephalographic predictors of outcome. *Intensive Care Med*. 2015;41(7):1264–72.

40. DB Seder, K Sunde, S Rubertsson et al. Neurologic outcomes and postresuscitation care of patients with myoclonus following cardiac arrest. *Crit Care Med*. 2015;43(5):965–72.

41. AR Panchal, JA Bartos, JG Cabañas et al. Part 3: Adult basic and advanced life support: 2020 American Heart Association Guidelines for Cardiopulmonary Resuscitation and Emergency Cardiovascular Care. *Circulation*. 2020;142(16 Suppl. 2):S366–468.

42. AO Rossetti, M Oddo, G Logroscino, and PW Kaplan. Prognostication after cardiac arrest and hypothermia: A prospective study. *Ann Neurol*. 2010;67(3):301–7.

43. H Søholm, TW Kjær, J Kjaergaard et al. Prognostic value of electroencephalography (EEG) after out-of-hospital cardiac arrest in successfully resuscitated patients used in daily clinical practice. *Resuscitation*. 2014;85(11):1580–5.

44. L Benarous, M Gavaret, M Soda Diop et al. Sources of interrater variability and prognostic value of standardized EEG features in post-anoxic coma after resuscitated cardiac arrest. *Clin Neurophysiol Pract*. 2019;4:20–6.

8

What Is the Best Long-Term Treatment Plan for Epilepsy Patients as an Outpatient?

This chapter applies information from previous chapters to specific concerns in long-term outpatient epilepsy practice.

Medication-Controlled Epilepsy

FIRST-TIME SEIZURE VERSUS EPILEPSY

The work-up and management of a first-time seizure was discussed thoroughly in Chapter 1. Since a high percentage of patients do not have a second seizure [1, 2], antiseizure medicine (ASM) treatment is indicated for patients meeting diagnostic criteria for epilepsy. Epilepsy is defined as any of the following [3]:

- Two or more unprovoked seizures >24 hours apart
- One unprovoked seizure and at least 60% probability of recurrent seizures
- Having an epilepsy syndrome.

The goal of treatment after initiation of an ASM is seizure freedom. About two-thirds of patients will be seizure free with medications alone [4].

KEEPING PATIENTS SEIZURE FREE

Antiseizure medicine compliance is the most important variable for maintaining seizure freedom. This must be a partnership between provider and patient. Providers can do their part through the following:

Minimizing ASM Dosing Complexity

Adherence decreases with dosing frequency increases, with 87% of patients adherent to daily, 81% to twice daily, 77% to three-times daily, and 39% to four-times daily [5]. A pillbox or smartphone apps may aid in adherence.

Minimizing ASM Side Effects and Interactions

This applies to both prescription and over-the-counter medications/supplements. Medication reconciliation should be performed at each visit, with patients providing updates of medications and supplements between visits if possible.

An exhaustive list of potential drug–drug interactions is too large to provide in this book; however, such searches are easily available online and through interaction application tools. Table 8.1 is a nonexhaustive

Table 8.1 Examples of medications and supplements that can affect seizure control

Common outpatient medications [6–9]	Supplements that lower ASM levels [10, 11]	Supplements that lower seizure threshold without affecting ASM [10, 11]
Bupropion	Ginkgo biloba	Ephedra
Clozapine	Borage	Eucalyptus
Tramadol	Shankhpushpi	Ginseng
Fluoroquinolone antibiotic	Yohimbine	Star fruit
		Wormwood

list of examples of prescriptions and supplements that can affect seizure control.

Lifestyle Management and Counseling

Sleep deprivation or increased alcohol intake (with likely accompanying poor sleep) are key exacerbators of epilepsy that are more patient controllable. Other precipitants like illness and stress are key to acknowledge and discuss with patients with the understanding that they are less directly modifiable [12, 13].

MANAGING COMORBIDITIES

Mental Health

Epilepsy is strongly associated with mental health comorbidities such as anxiety and depression [14]. Chapter 9 discusses the intersection of mental health and epilepsy independently due to the importance and frequency among epilepsy patients.

Osteoporosis, Fractures, Vitamin D, Calcium, and Bone Density Screening

Patients with epilepsy (PWE) are at increased risk for fractures [15], likely due to increased falls from seizures and decreased bone density from ASMs. Induction of cytochrome P450 enzymes by select ASMs as well as valproic acid appear to have the largest adverse effect on bone health [16, 17]. However, other ASMs also appear to affect bone health negatively [18].

Fracture risk increases with increasing age [19] and women appear to be most at risk [18]. It is reasonable to avoid enzyme-inducing ASMs or valproic acid when possible in these populations, though seizure freedom with one of those ASMs obviously provides sizable benefit.

No consensus guidelines exist for osteoporosis screening or preventative treatment for PWE. Vitamin D and calcium supplementation can be considered in all patients, most prominently in older patients and those taking enzyme-inducing ASMs or valproate. Vitamin D and calcium supplementation have been shown to increase bone mineral density in PWE, particularly when paired with risedronate [20]. It is reasonable to check vitamin D and calcium levels annually.

Bone mineral density screening is reasonable every three to five years for patients on enzyme inducers [21] or valproate. Patients who suffer any fracture should be evaluated. Screening can also be considered for older patients regardless of ASM and for vitamin D and calcium deficient patients. Consultation with an endocrinologist in uncertain situations can also be helpful.

Cardiac Risk

An increasingly recognized comorbidity in epilepsy is heart disease. It has been shown PWE may be at a 2.4-fold increased risk of heart disease [22] and a 2.9-fold increased risk of cardiac arrest [23]. Patients should be counseled on healthy diet and exercise. Coordination with primary care to ensure screening and treatment of any underlying heart disease is advisable.

ASM LEVEL MONITORING

The monitoring of ASM levels is useful only in specific settings. A randomized trial of drug monitoring versus clinical management in newer-generation ASMs in 2020 found no statistical difference in seizure or side effect frequency [24]. As such, routine drug-level monitoring with subsequent dosage adjustments is not recommended since routine clinical management is as effective as laboratory management for most situations. A 2008 practice guideline provides drug monitoring advice mostly applicable to older-generation ASMs [25]. Taken together, we recommend drug monitoring in the following clinical settings:

- Pregnancy (discussed in detail later in this chapter)
- When drug toxicity is suspected though clinical signs or symptoms are unclear, particularly with first-generation ASMs
- When adjusting ASM dosage in situations with increased pharmacokinetic variability such as chemotherapy, pregnancy, and so on
- When starting phenytoin, although we advise limiting outpatient use since other outpatient ASMs are simpler and safer to use.

It is reasonable to check drug levels for the following:

- To establish an individual therapeutic level with prolonged seizure freedom that can be used in comparison should the patient have a change in seizure control
- Verifying compliance – notably, this is done as a diagnostic step for uncontrolled epilepsy and should not assume negative intent on the patient's part.

Restrictions in Epilepsy

DRIVING

Lifestyle restrictions after breakthrough seizure have a major impact on patient quality of life. Of these restrictions, driving is the most notable, being of concern in up to ~65% of epilepsy patients [26].

- Strictly from a risk standpoint, the American Academy of Neurology supports a lifting of driving restrictions after a 3-month seizure-free period [27].
- From a legal standpoint, driving laws vary by state and country with seizure-free requirements ranging from 3 to 24 months.
- Providers should be familiar with local laws when counseling patients.
- More stringent restrictions apply to those seeking a commercial driver's license for interstate commerce, pilots, drivers of larger passenger vehicles/trains, and so on.

WORK AND EMPLOYMENT

- Patients with epilepsy should not be restricted from employment. Studies have shown that PWE have a mildly higher accident rate, though work injuries are typically mild and not related to seizures [28, 29].
- Epilepsy patients are protected from discrimination by the Americans with Disabilities Act and there are online resources for those working or seeking employment (US Equal Employment Opportunity Commission 2013).
- Patients with epilepsy are restricted from military service and rules for law enforcement vary by state [30].

OVERALL SEIZURE PRECAUTIONS/RESTRICTIONS

Patients should refrain from activities that could injure themselves or others if they were to have a seizure. Some common precautions include:
- Taking a shower instead of a bath
- Using the rear burners when cooking
- Avoiding heights when unsecured
- Avoiding swimming alone or without a life jacket
- Restricting power tool usage to those with safety features that prevent the machine from operating without the user actively holding a switch
- No scuba diving or sky diving.

ASM Discontinuation

DECIDING ON OFFERING A PATIENT AN ASM TAPER

Discontinuation of an ASM can be considered after a two-year seizure-free period [31]. The decision is not to be taken lightly as studies show about a third of patients relapse within two years after ASM withdrawal [32, 33]. *Thus, the question you should ask yourself is do you think the epilepsy is cured.*

The perceived risk of ASM taper can outweigh the benefit. Seizure recurrence can impact driving, employment, or even undue stress of worrying when/if another seizure will occur. Additionally, patients should be counseled that ~10% of patients who relapse after coming off ASM do not regain seizure freedom [34].

Specific factors that increase seizure relapse likelihood are the following [31]:

- Abnormal EEG at time of discontinuation
- Known etiology of epilepsy, including structural abnormalities on neuroimaging
- Focal seizures
- Older age at onset.

If a patient has two or more of these factors, patients should consider staying on ASM despite a two-year seizure-free period [31]. In essence, you do not think that their epilepsy is cured or remitted.

HOW TO TAPER AN ASM

A randomized trial in children found no difference in seizure relapse when comparing a 6-week to 9-month schedule [35]. Probably more influential in determining a taper schedule is the ASM itself; for instance, phenobarbital requires a prolonged taper. Still, most ASMs can be tapered on a shorter 6–8-week schedule. There is no clear direction on restrictions during ASM tapers. While a driving restriction is not legally required, it is worth individual discussions with patients on risks and benefits.

Special Consideration for Women with Epilepsy

This section will address the effects of estrogen and progesterone on epilepsy, ASM risk to the fetus and neurodevelopment, ASM management during childbearing years, and breastfeeding while taking ASMs.

HORMONAL EFFECTS AND CATAMENIAL EPILEPSY

Broadly, estrogen has been shown to be proconvulsant [36–38], whereas progesterone is anticonvulsant [39, 40]. The term catamenial epilepsy refers to cyclical hormone changes in the menstrual cycle that leads to cyclical worsening of seizure control [41]. A seizure diary can identify a catamenial pattern and suggest treatment strategies. In order of most common, three catamenial patterns surrounding the menstrual cycle have been identified:

- Perimenstrual (days –3 to 3) – caused by sudden drop in progesterone level
- Periovulatory (days 10 to –13) – caused by sudden increase in estrogen level
- Luteal (days 10 to 3 of the following cycle) in anovulatory cycles – caused by estrogen surge.

A trial of a benzodiazepine starting 2–4 days prior continued through the identified period may be beneficial [42].

While a randomized controlled trial showed exogenous progesterone to be ineffective as a whole, post hoc analysis suggested efficacy in women with three-times baseline seizure worsening during the perimenstrual period [43]. Acetazolamide may also be effective [44], though there have been no randomized trials to validate retrospective reports.

CONTRACEPTION

Enzyme-inducing ASMs lower the efficacy of hormonal contraception, both pills and depo implant [45–47]. When possible, enzyme-inducing ASMs should be avoided in women of childbearing age. If not possible, women should be counseled on the potentials for hormonal contraceptive failure. Since intrauterine devices are not affected by ASMs, they are considered the contraception method of choice for women with epilepsy [48]. Table 8.2 provides a list of ASMs that effect hormonal contraception.

Lastly, lamotrigine is an ASM of choice in women of childbearing age. It is critical to note oral contraceptives causes lowered lamotrigine levels due to increased metabolism [52]. Lamotrigine dosing may need to be increased when starting or lowered when stopping oral contraceptives.

PREGNANCY PLANNING

FOLATE CONSIDERATIONS

Many ASMs are associated with an increased risk of congenital malformations [53]. Folic acid supplementation has been shown to lower the risk of neural tube defects in the general population and in women with

Table 8.2 Medication effects of ASMs on hormonal contraception

Strong effect [49]	Weak effect [49–51]
Carbamazepine	Perampanel
Phenobarbital	Felbamate
Phenytoin	Topiramate
Oxcarbazepine	
Eslicarbazepine	
Clobazam	
Rufinamide	
Primidone	

epilepsy [54, 55]. We recommend 1 mg of folic acid daily in all women of childbearing age on ASMs. While common clinical practice to recommend 2–4 mg per day in women taking valproic acid or enzyme-inducing medications, there is limited data to support this recommendation.

CONGENITAL MALFORMATION RISK AND NEURODEVELOPMENTAL OUTCOMES

Certain ASMs impose a greater risk to the developing fetus and child. The baseline risk of major congenital malformation for women not on ASMs is ~2.4–2.6% [53, 56]. Table 8.3 contains a comparison of data for the risk with various ASMs as monotherapies. Levetiracetam and lamotrigine are ASMs of choice as they have not been found to significantly increase malformation risk [53, 56].

Table 8.3 Risk of major congenital malformations with different ASM monotherapies

	Cochrane Review – raw data, unweighted		International Registry of Antiepileptic Drugs and Pregnancy (EURAP)	
	Prevalence	95% CI	Prevalence	95% CI
Women with epilepsy not on ASM (baseline risk)	2.4% (32/1,310)	(1.7–3.4)		
Lamotrigine	2.3% (97/4,171)	(1.9–2.8)	2.9% (74/2,514)	(2.3–3.7)
Levetiracetam	1.7% (14/817)	(1.0–2.9)	2.8% (17/599)	(1.7–4.5)
Oxcarbazepine	2.5% (5/203)	(1.1–5.6)	3.0% (10/333)	(1.4–5.4)
Carbamazepine	3.6% (161/4,425)	(3.1–4.2)	5.5% (107/1,957)	(4.5–6.6)
Topiramate	4.0% (19/473)	(2.6–6.2)	3.9% (6/152)	(1.5–8.4)
Phenytoin	5.4% (60/1,117)	(4.2–6.9)	6.4% (8/125)	(2.8–12.2)
Phenobarbital	5.9% (43/730)	(4.4–7.8)	6.5% (19/294)	(4.2–9.9)
Valproic acid	8.7% (209/2,390)	(7.7–9.9)	10.3% (142/1,381)	(8.8–12.0)

Zonisamide, oxcarbazepine, and gabapentin have also not shown clear association with increased risk of major congenital malformations, although data are much more limited and should be interpreted with caution [53, 56, 57].

Valproic acid has the greatest malformation risk [53, 56, 57]. In addition, valproic acid has been shown to be associated with lower IQ in children exposed in utero [58]. Malformation risk also increases with polytherapy.

CHOOSING AN ASM FOR WOMEN IN CHILDBEARING AGE

It is common practice to preferentially use ASMs with lower risk to a fetus in women of childbearing age in the event of pregnancy. However, this should not absolutely contraindicate a higher-risk ASM more likely to make the woman seizure free. Time should be taken at each clinic visit to discuss any current or future plans for pregnancy. The risks associated with each ASM can be discussed individually so patients can make informed decisions.

If pregnancy is considered, it is highly recommended to transition off valproic acid if safe. It is reasonable to attempt a change in ASM for patients on carbamazepine, topiramate, phenobarbital, or phenytoin. Data are still limited for gabapentin and zonisamide, thus a change could be considered if on one of these medications. Any switch should be made to lamotrigine, levetiracetam, or oxcarbazepine.

ASM MANAGEMENT DURING PREGNANCY AND POSTNATALLY

Seizure frequency prior to pregnancy is the most important predictor of seizure frequency during pregnancy [59]. Pregnancy can increase

Table 8.4 Lamotrigine management in pregnancy

Prepregnancy	Prenatal	Postnatal

• Measure serum lamotrigine level to serve as a reference level
• If the patient is on hormonal-based contraception, recheck level two weeks after stopping contraception and lower lamotrigine dose if needed
• If the dose is adjusted, recheck in two weeks to ensure desired level has been achieved
	• Measure serum lamotrigine level every four weeks. May consider checking every two weeks in the last month of pregnancy
	  ◦ If the level is ≥ reference level, do not adjust dose
	  ◦ If the level is < reference level, increase dose by 20–25%
		• Measure serum lamotrigine level within one week of delivery (often on day of discharge)
		  ◦ If the level is > reference level, decrease dose by 20–25%
		  ◦ If the level is ≤ reference level, do not adjust the dose
		• Repeat level weekly and adjust accordingly
		  ◦ If the dose was increased ≥ four times during pregnancy, decrease dose by 20–25% on day 1 after delivery. After that, follow the aforementioned monitoring and adjustment schedule
		  ◦ If clinical signs of toxicity, level should be checked more frequently with dose adjusted accordingly

clearance of multiple ASMS and lead to breakthrough seizures [60]. The largest effect is seen on lamotrigine, our drug of choice in pregnancy [61].

Lamotrigine clearance increases during pregnancy and normalizes very quickly upon delivery. We utilize a published algorithm (Table 8.4) for lamotrigine management during pregnancy that uses a baseline prepregnancy level with levels checked every four weeks during pregnancy [62]:

A similar approach can be adapted to other ASMs, particularly levetiracetam and oxcarbazepine. Of note, the active metabolite of oxcarbazepine (10-monohydroxy-10, 11-dihydro-carbamazepine) is reduced in pregnancy and thus the level of the metabolite should be followed and not oxcarbazepine level [63].

BREASTFEEDING CONSIDERATIONS

Although all ASMs can be found in breast milk to varying degrees, benefits of breastfeeding generally outweigh the risks. Antiseizure medicine levels reached in the infant are typically low though depend on the concentration in the breast milk as well as absorption and clearance by the infant.

A prospective study of carbamazepine, carbamazepine-10–11-epoxide, levetiracetam, lamotrigine, oxcarbazepine, topiramate, valproate, and zonisamide found that ~49% of infants had concentrations less than the lower quantifiable limit. Those most detectable were lamotrigine and levetiracetam, which are considered safer medications [64]. An extension of the NEAD study also found a correlation between breastfeeding and higher IQ and verbal abilities at age 6 in children of women on one ASM (phenytoin, lamotrigine, valproate, or carbamazepine) [65].

Works Cited

1. Randomized clinical trial on the efficacy of antiepileptic drugs in reducing the risk of relapse after a first unprovoked tonic-clonic seizure: First Seizure Trial Group (FIR.S.T. Group). *Neurology*. 1993; 43 (3 pt. 1): 478–83.
2. A Marson, A Jacoby, A Johnson, L Kim, C Gamble, and D Chadwick. Immediate versus deferred antiepileptic drug treatment for early epilepsy and single seizures: A randomised controlled trial. *Lancet*. 2005;365(9476):2007–13.
3. RS Fisher, C Acevedo, A Arzimanoglou et al. ILAE official report: A practical clinical definition of epilepsy. *Epilepsia*. 2014;55(4):475–82.

4. Z Chen, MJ Brodie, D Liew, and P Kwan. Treatment outcomes in patients with newly diagnosed epilepsy treated with established and new antiepileptic drugs: A 30-year longitudinal cohort study. *JAMA Neurol*. 2018;75(3):279–86.

5. JA Cramer, RH Mattson, ML Prevey, RD Scheyer, and VL Ouellette. How often is medication taken as prescribed? A novel assessment technique. *JAMA*. 1989;261(22):3273–7.

6. C Johannessen Landmark, O Henning, and SI Johannessen. Proconvulsant effects of antidepressants: What is the current evidence? *Epilepsy Behav*. 2016;61:287–91.

7. AW Hitchings. Drugs that lower the seizure threshold. *Adverse Drug React Bull*. 2016;298(1):1151–4.

8. R Boostani and S Derakhshan. Tramadol induced seizure: A 3-year study. *Caspian J Intern Med*. 2012;3(3):484–7.

9. R Sutter, S Rüegg, and S Tschudin-Sutter. Seizures as adverse events of antibiotic drugs: A systematic review. *Neurology*. 2015;85(15):1332–41.

10. N Samuels, Y Finkelstein, SR Singer, and M Oberbaum. Herbal medicine and epilepsy: Proconvulsive effects and interactions with antiepileptic drugs. *Epilepsia*. 2008;49(3):373–80.

11. A Tyagi and N Delanty. Herbal remedies, dietary supplements, and seizures. *Epilepsia*. 2003;44(2):228–35.

12. MM Frucht, M Quigg, C Schwaner, and NB Fountain. Distribution of seizure precipitants among epilepsy syndromes. *Epilepsia*. 2000;41(12):1534–9.

13. M Wassenaar, DG Kasteleijn-Nolst Trenité, GJ de Haan, JA Carpay, and FS Leijten. Seizure precipitants in a community-based epilepsy cohort. *J Neurol*. 2014;261(4):717–24.

14. AJ Scott, L Sharpe, C Hunt, and M Gandy. Anxiety and depressive disorders in people with epilepsy: A meta-analysis. *Epilepsia*. 2017;58(6):973–82.

15. PC Souverein, DJ Webb, H Petri et al. Incidence of fractures among epilepsy patients: A population-based retrospective cohort study in the General Practice Research Database. *Epilepsia*. 2005;46(2):304–10.

16. JM Nicholas, L Ridsdale, MP Richardson, AP Grieve, and MC Gulliford. Fracture risk with use of liver enzyme inducing antiepileptic drugs in people with active epilepsy: Cohort study using the general practice research database. *Seizure*. 2013;22(1):37–42.

17. D Fan, J Miao, X Fan, Q Wang, and M Sun. Effects of valproic acid on bone mineral density and bone metabolism: A meta-analysis. *Seizure*. 2019;73:56–63.

18. PC Souverein, DJ Webb, JG Weil, TP van Staa, and AC Egberts. Use of antiepileptic drugs and risk of fractures: Case-control study among patients with epilepsy. *Neurology*. 2006;66(9):1318–24.

19. JA Kanis, F Borgstrom, C de Laet et al. Assessment of fracture risk. *Osteoporos Int.* 2005;16(6):581–9.

20. AA Lazzari, PM Dussault, M Thakore-James et al. Prevention of bone loss and vertebral fractures in patients with chronic epilepsy: Antiepileptic drug and osteoporosis prevention trial. *Epilepsia.* 2013;54(11):1997–2004.

21. ST Herman. Screening bone mineral density in epilepsy: A call to action, but what action? *Epilepsy Curr.* 2009;9(2):44–6.

22. M Zack and C Luncheon. Adults with an epilepsy history, notably those 45–64 years old or at the lowest income levels, more often report heart disease than adults without an epilepsy history. *Epilepsy Behav.* 2018;86:208–10.

23. A Bardai, RJ Lamberts, MT Blom et al. Epilepsy is a risk factor for sudden cardiac arrest in the general population. *PLoS One.* 2012;7(8):e42749.

24. I Aícua-Rapún, P André, AO Rossetti et al. Therapeutic drug monitoring of newer antiepileptic drugs: A randomized trial for dosage adjustment. *Ann Neurol.* 2020;87(1):22–9.

25. PN Patsalos, DJ Berry, BF Bourgeois et al. Antiepileptic drugs: Best practice guidelines for therapeutic drug monitoring: A position paper by the Subcommission on Therapeutic Drug Monitoring, ILAE Commission on Therapeutic Strategies. *Epilepsia.* 2008;49(7):1239–76.

26. F Gilliam, R Kuzniecky, E Faught et al. Patient-validated content of epilepsy-specific quality-of-life measurement. *Epilepsia.* 1997;38(2):233–6.

27. D Bacon, RS Fisher, JC Morris, M Rizzo, and MV Spanaki. American Academy of Neurology position statement on physician reporting of medical conditions that may affect driving competence. *Neurology.* 2007;68(15):1174–7.

28. AK Dasgupta, M Saunders, and DJ Dick. Epilepsy in the British Steel Corporation: An evaluation of sickness, accident, and work records. *Br J Ind Med.* 1982;39(2):145–8.

29. E Beghi and C Cornaggia. Morbidity and accidents in patients with epilepsy: Results of a European cohort study. *Epilepsia.* 2002;43(9):1076–83.

30. A Krumholz, JL Hopp, and AM Sanchez. Counseling epilepsy patients on driving and employment. *Neurol Clin.* 2016;34(2):427–42.

31. E Beghi, G Giussani, S Grosso et al. Withdrawal of antiepileptic drugs: Guidelines of the Italian League Against Epilepsy. *Epilepsia.* 2013;54(Suppl. 7):2–12.

32. Randomised study of antiepileptic drug withdrawal in patients in remission: Medical Research Council Antiepileptic Drug withdrawal Study Group. *Lancet.* 1991;337(8751):1175–80.

33. AT Berg and S Shinnar. Relapse following discontinuation of antiepileptic drugs: A meta-analysis. *Neurology.* 1994;44(4):601–8.

34. D Chadwick, J Taylor, and T Johnson. Outcomes after seizure recurrence in people with well-controlled epilepsy and the factors that influence it: The MRC Antiepileptic Drug withdrawal Group. *Epilepsia*. 1996;37(11):1043–50.

35. M Tennison, R Greenwood, D Lewis, and M Thorn. Discontinuing antiepileptic drugs in children with epilepsy: A comparison of a six-week and a nine-month taper period. *N Engl J Med*. 1994;330(20):1407–10.

36. SL Stitt and WJ Kinnard. The effect of certain progestins and estrogens on the threshold of electrically induced seizure patterns. *Neurology*. 1968;18(3):213–16.

37. DE Woolley and PS Timiras. The gonad–brain relationship: Effects of female sex hormones on electroshock convulsions in the rat. *Endocrinology*. 1962;70:196–209.

38. NG Weiland. Estradiol selectively regulates agonist binding sites on the N-methyl-D-aspartate receptor complex in the CA1 region of the hippocampus. *Endocrinology*. 1992;131(2):662–8.

39. DS Reddy. The role of neurosteroids in the pathophysiology and treatment of catamenial epilepsy. *Epilepsy Res*. 2009;85(1):1–30.

40. AG Herzog. Hormonal therapies: Progesterone. *Neurotherapeutics*. 2009;6(2):383–91.

41. AG Herzog. Catamenial epilepsy: Definition, prevalence pathophysiology and treatment. *Seizure*. 2008;17(2):151–9.

42. M Feely and J Gibson. Intermittent clobazam for catamenial epilepsy: Tolerance avoided. *J Neurol Neurosurg Psychiatry*. 1984;47(12):1279–82.

43. AG Herzog, KM Fowler, SD Smithson et al. Progesterone vs placebo therapy for women with epilepsy: A randomized clinical trial. *Neurology*. 2012;78(24):1959–66.

44. LL Lim, N Foldvary, E Mascha, and J Lee. Acetazolamide in women with catamenial epilepsy. *Epilepsia*. 2001;42(6):746–9.

45. AR Davis, CL Westhoff, and FZ Stanczyk. Carbamazepine coadministration with an oral contraceptive: Effects on steroid pharmacokinetics, ovulation, and bleeding. *Epilepsia*. 2011;52(2):243–7.

46. A Lazorwitz, A Davis, M Swartz, and M Guiahi. The effect of carbamazepine on etonogestrel concentrations in contraceptive implant users. *Contraception*. 2017;95(6):571–7.

47. M Haukkamaa. Contraception by Norplant subdermal capsules is not reliable in epileptic patients on anticonvulsant treatment. *Contraception*. 1986;33(6):559–65.

48. NJ Vélez-Ruiz and PB Pennell. Issues for women with epilepsy. *Neurol Clin*. 2016;34(2):411–25.

49. MJ Brodie, S Mintzer, AM Pack et al. Enzyme induction with antiepileptic drugs: Cause for concern? *Epilepsia*. 2013;54(1):11–27.

50. J Novy, LE Rothuizen, T Buclin, and AO Rossetti. Perampanel: A significant liver enzyme inducer in some patients? *Eur Neurol*. 2014;72(3–4):213–16.

51. MS Benedetti. Enzyme induction and inhibition by new antiepileptic drugs: A review of human studies. *Fundam Clin Pharmacol*. 2000;14(4):301–19.

52. J Christensen, V Petrenaite, J Atterman et al. Oral contraceptives induce lamotrigine metabolism: Evidence from a double-blind, placebo-controlled trial. *Epilepsia*. 2007;48(3):484–9.

53. J Weston, R Bromley, CF Jackson et al. Monotherapy treatment of epilepsy in pregnancy: Congenital malformation outcomes in the child. *Cochrane Database Syst Rev*. 2016;11(11):Cd010224.

54. Prevention of neural tube defects: Results of the Medical Research Council Vitamin Study: MRC Vitamin Study Research Group. *Lancet*. 1991;338(8760):131–7.

55. KJ Meador, GA Baker, N Browning et al. Fetal antiepileptic drug exposure and cognitive outcomes at age 6 years (NEAD study): A prospective observational study. *Lancet Neurol*. 2013;12(3):244–52.

56. AA Veroniki, E Cogo, P Rios et al. Comparative safety of anti-epileptic drugs during pregnancy: A systematic review and network meta-analysis of congenital malformations and prenatal outcomes. *BMC Med*. 2017;15(1):95.

57. T Tomson, D Battino, E Bonizzoni et al. Comparative risk of major congenital malformations with eight different antiepileptic drugs: A prospective cohort study of the EURAP registry. *Lancet Neurol*. 2018;17(6):530–8.

58. KJ Meador, GA Baker, N Browning et al. Fetal antiepileptic drug exposure and cognitive outcomes at age 6 years (NEAD study): A prospective observational study. *Lancet Neurol*. 2013;12(3):244–52.

59. SV Thomas, U Syam, and JS Devi. Predictors of seizures during pregnancy in women with epilepsy. *Epilepsia*. 2012;53(5):e85–8.

60. SI Patel and PB Pennell. Management of epilepsy during pregnancy: An update. *Ther Adv Neurol Disord*. 2016;9(2):118–29.

61. PB Pennell, L Peng, DJ Newport et al. Lamotrigine in pregnancy: Clearance, therapeutic drug monitoring, and seizure frequency. *Neurology*. 2008; 70 (22 pt. 2): 2130–6.

62. A Sabers. Algorithm for lamotrigine dose adjustment before, during, and after pregnancy. *Acta Neurol Scand*. 2012;126(1):e1–4.

63. V Petrenaite, A Sabers, and J Hansen-Schwartz. Seizure deterioration in women treated with oxcarbazepine during pregnancy. *Epilepsy Res*. 2009;84(2–3):245–9.

64. AK Birnbaum, KJ Meador, A Karanam et al. Antiepileptic drug exposure in infants of breastfeeding mothers with epilepsy. *JAMA Neurol*. 2020;77(4):441–50.

65. KJ Meador, GA Baker, N Browning et al. Breastfeeding in children of women taking antiepileptic drugs: Cognitive outcomes at age 6 years. *JAMA Pediatr*. 2014;168(8):729–36.

9

What to Do When Your Patient Fails Two Antiseizure Medicines
Managing Drug-Resistant Epilepsy as an Outpatient

Drug-resistant epilepsy (DRE) is defined as the failure of two adequately trialed and tolerated antiseizure medicines (ASMs) to achieve long-term seizure freedom [1]. Around a third of patients have DRE [2] and require different considerations in everyday management.

Medication Polytherapy

This topic was covered previously in Chapter 3. The highest proportion of patients become seizure free with their first ASM, with decreases in seizure-free rates after each subsequent ASM. In a 30-year cohort of patients with new onset epilepsy [2]

- 45.7% became seizure free with the first ASM
- 11.6% with the second ASMs in monotherapy
- 4.35% with the third ASMs in monotherapy
- Less than 1% of patients in the cohort became seizure free with subsequent ASMs in monotherapy.

At an earlier time point, the same cohort found only 6% of patients became seizure free with two ASM combination therapy, and less than 1% become seizure free on three or more ASMs [3]. Therefore, while ASM polytherapy has diminishing returns, a small portion of patients do find seizure freedom.

When considering polytherapy, the first thing to consider is does the patient meet the criteria for DRE. If the patient has DRE, a targeted approach to polytherapy can be made. Antiseizure medicines with different mechanisms of action should be chosen. For example, adding a GABAergic medicine to a sodium channel blocker allows for a multifaceted approach. Also, it is best to use ASMs without similar side effect profiles, as those side effects could be additive [4].

It should be equally stressed that DRE patients should be considered for epilepsy surgery evaluation, whether at your institution or with referral to an epilepsy center with surgical capabilities. An autoimmune etiology may also be considered and will be discussed in the following section.

Autoimmune Epilepsy

Epilepsy due to autoimmune etiology has become increasingly recognized in recent years and has been estimated to account for ~5–7% of all epilepsies [5]. Careful history can provide clues to an autoimmune etiology for patients with new onset epilepsy and DRE alike. Early recognition provides a better chance for response to treatment [6].

Some clinical features that should raise concern include rapidly DRE, rapidly progressive mental status changes, neuropsychiatric changes, viral prodrome, faciobrachial dystonic semiology, or a history of cancer [6, 7]. In the absence of a known etiology, patients with any of the previously mentioned clinical features should undergo autoimmune work-up including lumbar puncture and magnetic resonance imaging (MRI) (if not already obtained).

CSF studies may show signs of inflammation with lymphocytic predominant increase in WBC and/or an elevated protein >50 mg/dL [7]. An MRI brain without and with contrast may show T2-weighted fluid-attenuated inversion recovery (T2/FLAIR) hyperintensities in the mesial temporal lobe, which can be bilateral [7]. An MRI could also show multifocal T2/FLAIR hyperintensities consistent with demyelinating or inflammatory disease [7]. Conversely, if a DRE patient does not have clinical features suggesting an autoimmune etiology, expectedly those patients should not undergo an autoimmune evaluation.

Recently a predictive scoring system for autoantibody testing positivity, called the APE2 score, has been developed to help guide work-up consideration of an autoimmune etiology (Table 9.1). An APE2 score of ≥4 is 98% sensitive and 84% specific finding a neuronal specific antibody and should prompt neural autoantibody testing in both serum and CSF [7]:

Table 9.1 Antibody prevalence in epilepsy and encephalopathy (APE2 score)

New onset, rapidly progressive mental status changes developing over 1–6 weeks or new onset epilepsy (within one year of evaluation)	+1
Neuropsychiatric changes (agitation, aggression, emotional lability)	+1
Autonomic dysfunction (sustained atrial tachycardia, bradycardia, orthostatic hypotension, hyperhidrosis, labile blood pressure, ventricular tachycardia, asystole, GI dysmotility)	+1
Viral prodrome	+2
Fachiobrachial dystonic semiology	+3
Facial dyskinesia (in the absence of fachiobrachial dystonic seizures)	+2
Refractory epilepsy	+2
CSF consistent with inflammation (protein >50 mg/dL and/or lymphocytic pleocytosis >5 cells/mcl, if total number of CSF RBC < 1,000 cells/mcl)	+2
Brain MRI suggesting encephalitis (T2/FLAIR hyperintensity of one or both mesial temporal lobes, or multifocal hyperintensities in gray matter, white matter, or both compatible with demyelination or inflammation)	+2
Systemic cancer diagnosed within five years of onset of neurologic symptoms (excluding cutaneous squamous cell carcinoma, basal cell carcinoma, brain tumor, cancer with brain metastasis)	+2

Table from [7], some language adapted for space

Those highly suspected to have autoimmune epilepsy should undergo cancer screening, which can include:

- Computerized tomography (CT) chest, abdomen, and pelvis with contrast as the first evaluation [5]
- A scrotal ultrasound in men if CT is unrevealing
- A mammogram and transvaginal ultrasound in women if CT is unrevealing [5]
- If antibody testing reveals a neural specific antibody highly associated with cancer, a positron emission tomography (PET) scan may be considered [5].

Immunotherapy should be initiated as soon as possible if a neural specific antibody is found in the presence of suspected autoimmune epilepsy. With an APE2 score of ≥4 in a patient with DRE, it is reasonable to trial immunotherapy even with negative neural autoantibody testing [5].

Initial treatment options for autoimmune epilepsy include intravenous (IV) high-dose methylprednisolone, IV immunoglobulin, or plasma exchange [5]. There should also be strong emphasis on treatment of any underlying cancer that could be causal. Ongoing immunotherapy depends on the response to initial treatment trial and should be done with the assistance of a neuroimmunologist or epileptologist with training in this area.

Considering and Counseling Epilepsy Surgery

RESECTIVE SURGERY

There are clear data supporting epilepsy surgery in DRE patients. A 2003 joint practice parameter recommends that all patients with disabling focal seizures with impaired awareness who fail appropriate ASMs be referred to an epilepsy surgery center [8].

Review of the literature demonstrated that patients with mesial temporal lobe epilepsy (MTLE) become free of disabling seizures two-thirds of the time with anteromesial temporal lobe (ATL) resections. Additionally, in patients with neocortical epilepsy, ~50% become free of disabling seizures with resection, whereas 15% are not improved [8].

RANDOMIZED TRIALS FOR ATL

Two important randomized controlled trials (RCTs) of ATL for MTLE patients demonstrated superiority compared to continued medical therapy [9, 10]. The first trial in 2001 compared ATL to best medical treatment for 40 patients in each group [9]. The trial found 58% in the surgery group versus 8% in the medical group became free of disabling seizures. Even more significant was 38% in the surgery group versus 3% in the medical group became completely seizure free. There was also a significant improvement in quality of life in the surgery group. Twenty-two surgery patients (65%) had asymptomatic superior subquadrantic visual field deficits, a known risk [9].

Surgery caused adverse effects in four. One had a small thalamic infarct, causing focal sensory changes, one had a wound infection, and two had interfering verbal memory impairment. No patients died in the surgical group; one patient in the medical group died of sudden unexpected death in epilepsy [9].

A 2012 RCT evaluated "early" ATL in MTLE patients who had disabling seizures ≤2 years after becoming drug resistant [10]. There were 15 patients in the surgical group and 23 in the medical group. The trial found 73% in the surgery group versus 0% in the medical group were free of disabling seizures after two years follow-up. There was also a significant quality-of-life improvement in the surgery group.

BENEFIT OF EPILEPSY SURGERY CENTER REFERRAL

A referral to an epilepsy surgery center has benefits in addition to surgery. These centers often have advanced technologies that may not be cost effective in small hospitals. This includes 3 Tesla (3T) MRI, functional MRI (fMRI), single photon emission computed tomography (SPECT), and intracranial electroencephalography (EEG). Centers commonly have additional psychosocial support such as social workers and comprehensive mental health specifically geared toward epilepsy patients.

Epilepsy surgery is a major decision and thus should not be left to only one physician. A multidisciplinary presurgical conference brings together epileptologists, neurosurgeons, neuropsychologists, neuroradiologists, and nuclear medicine radiologists to discuss each case prior to surgery. Each patient's epilepsy history, seizure semiology, relevant medical history, interictal and ictal EEG data, neuroimaging, and neuropsychology testing results are presented.

After review of that data, each physician provides input in their respective fields as it pertains to the patient. For instance, epileptologists may discuss pertinent semiology or EEG findings while neurosurgeons provide input as to possible surgical techniques. Afterward the managing epileptologist and neurosurgeon relay a consensus recommendation to the patient.

Neurostimulators

MRI CONSIDERATIONS FOR PATIENTS WITH A NEUROSTIMULATOR

Patients should be fully evaluated for resective surgeries prior to neurostimulator placement due to MRI restrictions caused by the neurostimulator. An increase in seizure frequency after MRI should prompt you to interrogate the device to ensure settings were restored properly.

MRI CONSIDERATIONS FOR VAGUS NERVE STIMULATION

At the time of this writing, all vagus nerve stimulation (VNS) devices are MRI conditional [11]. Magnetic resonance imaging settings are dependent on the model number and the location of the generator in the chest. While a 3T MRI is possible, there are limitations to the radiofrequency coils or time limit, which may lead to poorer-quality images [11].

To obtain the MRI, an imaging technician interrogates the device prior to MRI and notes the settings. The stimulation current parameter will be set to zero for the duration of the MRI and then returned to the original settings after MRI completion.

MRI CONSIDERATIONS FOR DEEP BRAIN STIMULATION

Obtaining an MRI for deep brain stimulation (DBS) patients is more restrictive. Only the newest model is 3T conditional [12]. An online worksheet from Medtronic can assess MRI eligibility. To obtain the MRI itself, the DBS should be placed into MRI mode and then restored to baseline settings following MRI completion [12].

MRI CONSIDERATIONS FOR RESPONSIVE NEUROSTIMULATION

Responsive neurostimulation (RNS) is the most MRI restrictive. Model RNS-300M is not MRI safe [13]. Model RNS-320 is MRI conditional with

1.5T but not 3T MRI [13]. The device should be placed in MRI mode
immediately prior to MRI then restored afterward [13].

VNS OUTCOMES

Vagus nerve stimulation therapy is a palliative consideration for DRE.
Compared to resective surgery, VNS palliation is inferior; thus, VNS
should be reserved only for patients with DRE who are not candidates for
resective surgery. Two RCTs had the following mean seizure *reduction* for
treatment versus control:

- 24.5 versus 6.1% seizure reduction in treatment versus control [14]
- 28 versus 15% seizure reduction in treatment versus control [15].

Additional studies report ~50% of patients have a 50% reduction in
seizures [16, 17].

VNS EVERYDAY USE

Vagus nerve stimulation may be turned on 2 weeks after implantation
after assessing for proper wound healing. Initial settings are listed in
Table 9.2 [18–20]. Auto stim mode (if applicable to patient's model) and
magnet mode output current should be kept slightly higher than normal
mode, often 0.25 mA higher.

After initiation of VNS, the output current should be increased by
0.25 mA every 2 weeks as tolerated until reaching goal settings or adequate
response if reached at a lower output than the goal [19]. An increase of
0.5 mA at once may be possible if the patient tolerates the change.

Tolerability should be assessed for any change prior to leaving the
office. If there has been no benefit after reaching goal settings, a slow
increase in duty cycle can be attempted by slightly decreasing the OFF
stimulation time; however, this should be done in consultation with an
epileptologist, with specific parameters are beyond the scope of this book.

Table 9.2 VNS settings

	Initial settings	Goal settings
Normal mode		
Output current	0.25 mA	1–1.75 mA
Signal frequency	30 Hz	30 Hz
Pulse width	250–500 microseconds	250–500 microseconds
Signal ON time	30 seconds	30 seconds
Signal OFF time	5 minutes	5 minutes
Auto stim mode		
Output current	0.375 mA	1.125–1.875 mA
Pulse width	250–500 microseconds	250–500 microseconds
ON time	60 seconds	60 seconds
Magnet mode		
Output current	0.5 mA	1.25–2 mA
Pulse width	500 microseconds[a]	500 microseconds[a]
ON time	60 seconds	60 seconds

[a] Ensure patient can tolerate 500-microsecond pulse width magnet if using a lower setting on normal mode

Magnet mode is used for abortive therapy during seizures. Patients or family members can be trained to swipe the magnet over their VNS generator at seizure onset.

Newer features like Auto stim mode sends an additional stimulation in response to a prespecified increase in heart rate. Tachycardia detection must be enabled for Auto stim to work. The initial threshold setting should be 20% but can be increased if not tolerated or too many nonseizure-related stimulations are occurring, that is, during exercise or other activities [18].

VNS

Common side effects with VNS include voice changes, cough, local pain or paresthesias, and dyspnea that commonly occur during stimulation, often related to stimulation intensity [15, 21–23]. If a patient has intolerable side effects at a particular output current, the pulse width can be lowered to 250 microseconds (if at 500 microseconds currently) or the current can be reduced to give a longer period of adjustment before attempting the increase. Patients with VNS should also be monitored for sleep apnea as VNS can worsen or cause sleep apnea in some patients [24–26].

DBS AND RNS

Deep brain stimulation for epilepsy was FDA approved in 2018. It contrasts to the peripheral nerve stimulation of VNS with stimulation of the bilateral anterior nucleus of the thalamus for DBS. The initial DBS RCT showed a median seizure frequency reduction of 40.4% in the stimulation group versus 14.5% in the control group at 3 months [27]. Deep brain stimulation appears to become more effective with time as median reduction in seizure frequency in the unblinded portion of the study rose to 50–69% at 5 years depending on analysis types [28]. Patients should be monitored for signs of depression and memory impairment [27].

Responsive neurostimulation was FDA approved in 2013 with a substantially different mechanism. Responsive neurostimulation only stimulates when the device detects a seizure (hence it is responsive) with stimulation directed at the seizure onset area. For this reason, the seizure focus must be identified, with only one or two foci able to be stimulated. The initial RNS RCT showed a median reduction in seizure frequency of 37.9% in the stimulation group versus 17.3% in the control group at 3 months [29]. Responsive neurostimulation becomes more effective with time as median seizure frequency reduction in an unblinded continuation study was ~<60% at 3 years, ~>60% at 5 years, and 70–75% at 9 years depending on the type of analysis [30].

Deep brain stimulation and RNS can be valuable tools in the treatment of epilepsy when resective surgery is not an option or if patients do not wish to undergo resective surgery. Programming of these devices is beyond the scope of this book and should be done so by or in consultation with an epileptologist.

Brief Overview of Intracranial EEG

Intracranial EEG is necessary when noninvasive EEG, neuroimaging, and clinical data are unable to clearly identify the exact epileptogenic zone. Two types of intracranial EEG are available, subdural electrodes (SDEs) and stereoelectroencephalography (sEEG).

Subdural electrodes come in the form of grids or strips of electrodes. Subdural electrodes most commonly require a craniotomy for direct placement, though small strips can at times be placed through a burr hole [31]. They may be preferred when sampling a continuous area of neocortex or an eloquent area where careful cortical mapping can delineate functional tissue [32]. Stereoelectroencephalography involves drilling small holes in the skull and stereotactic placement of depth electrodes into a predefined area of gray matter with the guidance of special frames or robot assisted [33]. Stereoelectroencephalography is preferred when sampling of deep regions such as limbic areas and regions that are not spatially continuous [34]. It has the distinct advantage of shorter recovery time and decreased perioperative pain by avoiding a craniotomy [32]. It also has lower overall complication rates (1.3%) [35] than SDEs (3.5%) [36]. Introduction of sEEG has been shown to expand surgical epilepsy programs [37].

Brief Overview of Minimally Invasive Surgical Therapies

Resective surgery is the gold standard in epilepsy care, however, there are several minimally invasive procedures that can be utilized. These methods may be preferred at times for their faster recovery, albeit with

Table 9.3 Metaanalysis of MTLE surgical outcomes

	Engel 1 outcome	Major complication rate
ATL	69% (1032/1,504)	10.9%
Open selective amygdalohippocampectomy	66% (887/1,326)	7.4%
Laser interstitial thermal therapy	57% (315/554)	3.8%
Radiofrequency ablation	44% (54/123)	3.7%

the trade of less efficacy for seizure control. A recent metaanalysis' findings are summarized in Table 9.3 [38].

Laser interstitial thermal therapy (LITT) involves placement of a laser fiber directly into the epileptogenic region and subsequent ablation utilizing MRI thermometry for ongoing feedback throughout the procedure [39]. It has the advantage of lower morbidity and shorter hospitalizations than ATL [38, 40].

Laser interstitial thermal therapy's efficacy has been most examined in MTLE LITT cohorts. A prospective multicenter cohort reported an Engel 1 outcome in 70.8% of MTLE patients [41]. A retrospective multicenter cohort reported 58% Engel 1 outcomes at 1 year [42]. Single-institution series report 38–76% seizure-free rates at 1 year [39, 43–48].

Outcomes for non-MTLE LITT are less well studied. A prospective multicenter cohort reported Engel 1 outcomes in 55.6% of patients (10/18) [41], while a single-center cohort reported Engel 1 outcomes for 44% of patients (14/32) [49]. A pediatric cohort reported Engel 1 outcomes in 41% of patients (7/17) [50].

Radiofrequency ablation (RFA) is a procedure with a similar concept to LITT in that it results in thermal destruction of the tissue, though RFA uses radiofrequency current [51]. An RFA probe can be inserted into the target for treatment, but RFA can also be performed using sEEG contacts during intracranial EEG assessment [51]. The latter method has yielded ~11%

seizure free rates in various small studies, though has been up to 67% when treating epilepsy due to abnormalities of cortical development [52–55].

Stereotactic radiosurgery (SRS) is a procedure that utilizes targeted radiation to treat the epileptogenic lesion without the need of any intracranial manipulation. A 2018 RCT of SRS versus ATL for the treatment of MTLE found SRS less effective at 52% seizure free versus 78% seizure free with ATL [56]. Though less effective, it is minimally invasive and has shown slightly better neuropsychological outcomes than ATL [57].

Brief Overview of Ketogenic Diet

For patients who are not surgical candidates, a ketogenic diet (KD) can be considered. The goal of a KD is to induce a dietary state for which the brain shifts from glucose to ketones as the primary fuel source. The general principle is a regimented high fat, low carbohydrate diet. Given these dietary restrictions, it is typically not well tolerated in adults, with many studies showing large withdrawals or losses to follow-up [58].

Still, in very motivated patients or those utilizing tube feedings, it is a reasonable option. A 2018 metaanalysis found ~50% of participants had a 50% reduction in seizures [58]. There are four main KD therapies [59]:

(1) Traditional KD
(2) Medium-chain triglyceride diet
(3) Modified Atkins diet
(4) Low glycemic index diet.

Each diet has its own benefits with varying tolerability, as some are stricter than others. If considering KD, consultation with a dietitian is mandatory. That consultation can help decide if and which type of KD is right for each patient. Regular follow-up visits with the dietitian help ensure proper nutrition.

Baseline height, weight, and BMI should be obtained prior to initiation. Initial lab work should be obtained then followed every

Table 9.4 Evaluations for a KD [59, 64]

Prior to initiation	Every 3 months[a]	Annually or less often
CMP	CMP	Zinc
CBC with differential	CBC with Diff	Selenium
Calcium	Calcium	Bone density scan
Magnesium	Magnesium	(every 2 years)
Phosphate	Phosphate	
Fasting lipid profile	Fasting lipid profile	
Serum acylcarnitine profile	Serum acylcarnitine profile	
Vitamin D level	Vitamin D level	
Urine pregnancy test (women)	Urinalysis	
Urinalysis	Urine calcium and chromium	
Urine calcium and chromium		
Urine organic acids[b]		
Serum amino acids[b]		
Echocardiogram		

a. After one year, it is reasonable to decrease evaluations to every 6 months
b. Optional in adults, check in patient's suspected of having a metabolic disorder

3 months for the first year followed by every 6 months [59]. Table 9.4 contains recommended lab work.

Patients should take a multivitamin that includes minerals, calcium, and vitamin D [59]. Further supplementation may be needed based on laboratory evaluations and other needs as determined by the dietician.

KD SIDE EFFECTS

The most common side effects are manageable gastrointestinal symptoms such as constipation, vomiting, and abdominal pain [59]. Hyperlipidemia is also very common, but may normalize with time [60]. Kidney stones are common thus there should be a low threshold for ultrasound [58]. Cardiomyopathy and/or QT prolongation have also been reported [61–63].

Works Cited

1. P Kwan, A Arzimanoglou, AT Berg et al. Definition of drug resistant epilepsy: Consensus proposal by the ad hoc Task Force of the ILAE Commission on Therapeutic Strategies. *Epilepsia*. 2010;51(6):1069–77.

2. Z Chen, MJ Brodie, D Liew, and P Kwan. Treatment outcomes in patients with newly diagnosed epilepsy treated with established and new antiepileptic drugs: A 30-year longitudinal cohort study. *JAMA Neurol*. 2018;75(3):279–86.

3. MJ Brodie, SJ Barry, GA Bamagous, JD Norrie, and P Kwan. Patterns of treatment response in newly diagnosed epilepsy. *Neurology*. 2012;78(20):1548–54.

4. EK St. Louis. Truly "rational" polytherapy: Maximizing efficacy and minimizing drug interactions, drug load, and adverse effects. *Curr Neuropharmacol*. 2009;7(2):96–105.

5. KS Husari and D Dubey. Autoimmune epilepsy. *Neurotherapeutics*. 2019;16(3):685–702.

6. D Dubey, J Singh, JW Britton et al. Predictive models in the diagnosis and treatment of autoimmune epilepsy. *Epilepsia*. 2017;58(7):1181–9.

7. D Dubey, N Kothapalli, A McKeon et al. Predictors of neural-specific autoantibodies and immunotherapy response in patients with cognitive dysfunction. *J Neuroimmunol*. 2018;323:62–72.

8. J Engel, Jr., S Wiebe, J French et al. Practice parameter: Temporal lobe and localized neocortical resections for epilepsy: Report of the Quality Standards Subcommittee of the American Academy of Neurology, in association with the American Epilepsy Society and the American Association of Neurological Surgeons. *Neurology*. 2003;60(4):538–47.

9. S Wiebe, WT Blume, JP Girvin, and M Eliasziw. A randomized, controlled trial of surgery for temporal-lobe epilepsy. *N Engl J Med*. 2001;345(5):311–18.

10. J Engel, Jr., MP McDermott, S Wiebe et al. Early surgical therapy for drug-resistant temporal lobe epilepsy: A randomized trial. *JAMA*. 2012;307(9):922–30.

11. Livanova, PLC. MRI with the VNS Therapy System. 26–0010–0300. London: Livanova, PLC. October 2019.

12. Medtronic, Inc. MRI Guidelines for Medtronic Deep Brain Stimulation Systems. M929535A074 Rev. B. Minneapolis, MN: Medtronic, Inc. January 7, 2021.

13. Neuropace, Inc. MRI Guidelines for the RNS System. DN 1017451 Rev. 6. Mountain View, CA: Neuropace, Inc. February 2020.

14. E Ben-Menachem, R Mañon-Espaillat, R Ristanovic et al. Vagus nerve stimulation for treatment of partial seizures: 1. A controlled study of effect on seizures. First International Vagus Nerve Stimulation Study Group. *Epilepsia*. 1994;35(3):616–26.

15. A Handforth, CM DeGiorgio, SC Schachter et al. Vagus nerve stimulation therapy for partial-onset seizures: A randomized active-control trial. *Neurology*. 1998;51(1):48–55.

16. K Kawai, T Tanaka, H Baba et al. Outcome of vagus nerve stimulation for drug-resistant epilepsy: The first three years of a prospective Japanese registry. *Epileptic Disord*. 2017;19(3):327–38.

17. MA García-Pallero, E García-Navarrete, CV Torres et al. Effectiveness of vagal nerve stimulation in medication-resistant epilepsy: Comparison between patients with and without medication changes. *Acta Neurochir (Wien)*. 2017;159(1):131–6.

18. RS Fisher, P Afra, M Macken et al. Automatic vagus nerve stimulation triggered by ictal tachycardia: Clinical outcomes and device performance – The U.S. E-37 Trial. *Neuromodulation*. 2016;19(2):188–95.

19. C Heck, SL Helmers, and CM DeGiorgio. Vagus nerve stimulation therapy, epilepsy, and device parameters: Scientific basis and recommendations for use. *Neurology*. 2002;59(6 suppl. 4):S31–7.

20. SL Helmers, J Begnaud, A Cowley et al. Application of a computational model of vagus nerve stimulation. *Acta Neurol Scand*. 2012;126(5):336–43.

21. A randomized controlled trial of chronic vagus nerve stimulation for treatment of medically intractable seizures: The Vagus Nerve Stimulation Study Group. *Neurology*. 1995;45(2):224–30.

22. RE Ramsay, BM Uthman, LE Augustinsson et al. Vagus nerve stimulation for treatment of partial seizures: 2. Safety, side effects, and tolerability. First International Vagus Nerve Stimulation Study Group. *Epilepsia*. 1994;35(3):627–36.

23. ST Aaronson, LL Carpenter, CR Conway et al. Vagus nerve stimulation therapy randomized to different amounts of electrical charge for treatment-resistant depression: Acute and chronic effects. *Brain Stimul*. 2013;6(4):631–40.

24. BA Malow, J Edwards, M Marzec, O Sagher, and G Fromes. Effects of vagus nerve stimulation on respiration during sleep: A pilot study. *Neurology*. 2000;55(10):1450–4.

25. M Marzec, J Edwards, O Sagher, G Fromes, and BA Malow. Effects of vagus nerve stimulation on sleep-related breathing in epilepsy patients. *Epilepsia*. 2003;44(7):930–5.

26. T Hsieh, M Chen, A McAfee, and Y Kifle. Sleep-related breathing disorder in children with vagal nerve stimulators. *Pediatr Neurol*. 2008;38(2):99–103.

27. R Fisher, V Salanova, T Witt et al. Electrical stimulation of the anterior nucleus of thalamus for treatment of refractory epilepsy. *Epilepsia*. 2010;51(5):899–908.

28. V Salanova, T Witt, R Worth et al. Long-term efficacy and safety of thalamic stimulation for drug-resistant partial epilepsy. *Neurology*. 2015;84(10):1017–25.

29. MJ Morrell. Responsive cortical stimulation for the treatment of medically intractable partial epilepsy. *Neurology*. 2011;77(13):1295–304.

30. DR Nair, KD Laxer, PB Weber et al. Nine-year prospective efficacy and safety of brain-responsive neurostimulation for focal epilepsy. *Neurology*. 2020;95(9):e1244–56.

31. Y Nagahama, AJ Schmitt, D Nakagawa et al. Intracranial EEG for seizure focus localization: Evolving techniques, outcomes, complications, and utility of combining surface and depth electrodes. *J Neurosurg*. 2018;130(4):1–13.

32. DJ Englot. A modern epilepsy surgery treatment algorithm: Incorporating traditional and emerging technologies. *Epilepsy Behav*. 2018;80:68–74.

33. JS Katz and TJ Abel. Stereoelectroencephalography versus subdural electrodes for localization of the epileptogenic zone: What is the evidence? *Neurotherapeutics*. 2019;16(1):59–66.

34. JA Gonzalez-Martinez. The stereo-electroencephalography: The epileptogenic zone. *J Clin Neurophysiol*. 2016;33(6):522–9.

35. JP Mullin, M Shriver, S Alomar et al. Is SEEG safe? A systematic review and meta-analysis of stereo-electroencephalography-related complications. *Epilepsia*. 2016;57(3):386–401.

36. R Arya, FT Mangano, PS Horn et al. Adverse events related to extraoperative invasive EEG monitoring with subdural grid electrodes: A systematic review and meta-analysis. *Epilepsia*. 2013;54(5):828–39.

37. C Miller, B Schatmeyer, P Landazuri et al. sEEG for expansion of a surgical epilepsy program: Safety and efficacy in 152 consecutive cases. *Epilepsia Open*. 2021;6(4):694–702.

38. K Kohlhase, JP Zöllner, N Tandon, A Strzelczyk, and F Rosenow. Comparison of minimally invasive and traditional surgical approaches for refractory mesial temporal lobe epilepsy: A systematic review and meta-analysis of outcomes. *Epilepsia*. 2021;62(4):831–45.

39. JT Willie, NG Laxpati, DL Drane et al. Real-time magnetic resonance-guided stereotactic laser amygdalohippocampotomy for mesial temporal lobe epilepsy. *Neurosurgery*. 2014;74(6):569–84; discussion 84–5.

40. M Sharma, T Ball, A Alhourani et al. Inverse national trends of laser interstitial thermal therapy and open surgical procedures for refractory epilepsy: A nationwide inpatient sample-based propensity score matching analysis. *Neurosurg Focus*. 2020;48(4):E11.

41. P Landazuri, J Shih, E Leuthardt et al. A prospective multicenter study of laser ablation for drug resistant epilepsy: One year outcomes. *Epilepsy Res*. 2020;167:106473.

42. C Wu, WJ Jermakowicz, S Chakravorti et al. Effects of surgical targeting in laser interstitial thermal therapy for mesial temporal lobe epilepsy: A multicenter study of 234 patients. *Epilepsia*. 2019;60(6):1171–83.

43. RE Gross, MA Stern, JT Willie et al. Stereotactic laser amygdalohippocampotomy for mesial temporal lobe epilepsy. *Ann Neurol*. 2018;83(3):575–87.

44. WJ Jermakowicz, AM Kanner, S Sur et al. Laser thermal ablation for mesiotemporal epilepsy: Analysis of ablation volumes and trajectories. *Epilepsia*. 2017;58(5):801–10.

45. S Le, AL Ho, RS Fisher et al. Laser interstitial thermal therapy (LITT): Seizure outcomes for refractory mesial temporal lobe epilepsy. *Epilepsy Behav*. 2018;89:37–41.

46. C Donos, J Breier, E Friedman et al. Laser ablation for mesial temporal lobe epilepsy: Surgical and cognitive outcomes with and without mesial temporal sclerosis. *Epilepsia*. 2018;59(7):1421–32.

47. JY Kang, C Wu, J Tracy et al. Laser interstitial thermal therapy for medically intractable mesial temporal lobe epilepsy. *Epilepsia*. 2016;57(2):325–34.

48. BE Youngerman, JY Oh, D Anbarasan et al. Laser ablation is effective for temporal lobe epilepsy with and without mesial temporal sclerosis if hippocampal seizure onsets are localized by stereoelectroencephalography. *Epilepsia*. 2018;59(3):595–606.

49. K Gupta, B Cabaniss, A Kheder et al. Stereotactic MRI-guided laser interstitial thermal therapy for extratemporal lobe epilepsy. *Epilepsia*. 2020;61(8):1723–34.

50. EC Lewis, AG Weil, M Duchowny et al. MR-guided laser interstitial thermal therapy for pediatric drug-resistant lesional epilepsy. *Epilepsia*. 2015;56(10):1590–8.

51. J Voges, L Büntjen, and FC Schmitt. Radiofrequency-thermoablation: General principle, historical overview and modern applications for epilepsy. *Epilepsy Res*. 2018;142:113–16.

52. P Bourdillon, J Isnard, H Catenoix et al. Stereo electroencephalography-guided radiofrequency thermocoagulation (SEEG-guided RF-TC) in drug-resistant focal epilepsy: Results from a 10-year experience. *Epilepsia*. 2017;58(1):85–93.

53. M Cossu, D Fuschillo, G Casaceli et al. Stereoelectroencephalography-guided radiofrequency thermocoagulation in the epileptogenic zone: A retrospective study on 89 cases. *J Neurosurg*. 2015;123(6):1358–67.

54. H Catenoix, P Bourdillon, M Guénot, and J Isnard. The combination of stereo-EEG and radiofrequency ablation. *Epilepsy Res*. 2018;142:117–20.

55. H Catenoix, F Mauguière, M Guénot et al. SEEG-guided thermocoagulations: A palliative treatment of nonoperable partial epilepsies. *Neurology*. 2008;71(21):1719–26.

56. NM Barbaro, M Quigg, MM Ward et al. Radiosurgery versus open surgery for mesial temporal lobe epilepsy: The randomized, controlled ROSE trial. *Epilepsia*. 2018;59(6):1198–207.

57. M Quigg, DK Broshek, NM Barbaro et al. Neuropsychological outcomes after Gamma Knife radiosurgery for mesial temporal lobe epilepsy: A prospective multicenter study. *Epilepsia*. 2011;52(5):909–16.

58. H Liu, Y Yang, Y Wang et al. Ketogenic diet for treatment of intractable epilepsy in adults: A meta-analysis of observational studies. *Epilepsia Open*. 2018;3(1):9–17.

59. EH Kossoff, BA Zupec-Kania, S Auvin et al. Optimal clinical management of children receiving dietary therapies for epilepsy: Updated recommendations of the International Ketogenic Diet Study Group. *Epilepsia Open*. 2018;3(2):175–92.

60. DK Groesbeck, RM Bluml, and EH Kossoff. Long-term use of the ketogenic diet in the treatment of epilepsy. *Dev Med Child Neurol*. 2006;48(12):978–81.

61. IM Bank, SD Shemie, B Rosenblatt, C Bernard, and AS Mackie. Sudden cardiac death in association with the ketogenic diet. *Pediatr Neurol*. 2008;39(6):429–31.

62. TH Best, DN Franz, DL Gilbert, DP Nelson, and MR Epstein. Cardiac complications in pediatric patients on the ketogenic diet. *Neurology*. 2000;54(12):2328–30.

63. S Sharma and S Gulati. The ketogenic diet and the QT interval. *J Clin Neurosci*. 2012;19(1):181–2.

64. MC Cervenka and EH Kossoff. Dietary treatment of intractable epilepsy. *Continuum (Minneapolis, Minn)*. 2013;19(3 Epilepsy):756–66.

10

Nonepileptic Events and General Psychiatric Care for Epilepsy Patients

Nonepileptic Events

A nonepileptic event (NEE) is defined as a paroxysmal change in behavior or consciousness, at times with associated abnormal movements, sensations, or experience, in the absence of electrophysiological changes that accompany an epileptic seizure, and without evidence to suggest another somatic cause [1]. Many names have been used previously including pseudoseizure, psychogenic seizure, psychogenic nonepileptic seizure (PNES), nonepileptic seizure, among others.

"Pseudo" can certainly give the implication of "not real." This can unfortunately lead to dismissive behaviors from providers. "Psychogenic" can be misinterpreted by the patient as if you think that they are "crazy." "Seizure" could lead to unintended treatment as an epileptic seizure. For these reasons, we prefer the term nonepileptic events or attacks.

Nonepileptic events are commonly encountered in epilepsy practice. There is an estimated prevalence of up to 33/100,000 [2] and annual incidence of ~5/100,000 [3]. There is about a 3 to 1 ratio of women to men [4].

Nonepileptic events can be devastating for patients. They can incur worse quality of life than that of epilepsy [5]. One study demonstrated up to 87% of patients with NEEs are unemployed and 50% on disability. The study also showed that 16% of patients reported previous admission to an

ICU and 59% reported more than two hospitalizations [6]. The estimated lifetime costs in 2004 for these patients reaches US$100,000 [7].

DIAGNOSIS

Early diagnosis and treatment are important in improving outcomes [6, 8]. Unfortunately, NEEs are often mistaken for epilepsy, with an average delay in diagnosis of seven to eight years [9, 10]. During this time, patients are subjected to many unnecessary trials of antiseizure medicines (ASMs) [10].

Like epilepsy, diagnosis of NEEs starts with a good history. There are certain semiologic features and other clinical factors that are more common with NEEs versus epilepsy seizures (ESs) (Table 10.1). If possible, patients should be encouraged to have someone take a video of their event for review.

Features suggestive of NEEs include asynchronous or nonrhythmic clonic movements, fluctuating course, preserved awareness with

Table 10.1 Common clinical features of NEEs and ESs

NEEs	ESs
Asynchronous or nonrhythmic clonic movements	Synchronous and rhythmic clonic movements
Preserved awareness with bilateral movements	Occurrence from sleep
Eye fluttering	Eye opening at onset
Eyes closed at onset	Consistent stereotypy
Pelvic thrusting	
Prolonged events, consistently >5 minutes	
Intensify or alleviate with suggestion	
Fluctuating course ("start stop quality")	
Side-to-side movements	

bilateral movements, eye flutter, eyes closed, side-to-side head or body movements, and pelvic thrusting [11, 12]. Consistently prolonged events should also raise suspicion for NEEs as the majority of ESs stop within 2 minutes [13–15].

Features that can suggest an ES include eyes opening at onset, synchronous movements, and occurrence out of sleep [11, 12, 16]. Occurrence out of sleep is most valuable in an epilepsy monitoring unit (EMU) setting when sleep can be confirmed with an electroencephalogram (EEG). Patients with NEEs can have "pseudosleep," which would be indistinguishable from physiologic sleep without EEG [17].

It is reasonable to make the NEE diagnosis based on history. The Rule of 2s has an 85% positive predictive value for NEEs: 2 normal EEGs without previous EEGs showing epileptiform activity, 2 events or more weekly, and refractory to at least 2 ASMs [18]. When the NEE diagnosis is made, you can trial cognitive behavioral therapy (CBT) in patients with multiple nonepileptic features and a normal routine EEG. This is especially true in patients with infrequent events and those who respond positively to the delivery of diagnosis.

Any discrepancy in the clinical features, continued events despite CBT, or patient hesitancy in the acceptance of the NEE diagnosis should prompt video EEG, as the gold standard for NEE diagnosis remains video EEG [12].

A routine EEG with video may be sufficient in patients with very frequent events or whom have a trigger than can be recreated in the lab. An ambulatory video EEG may be utilized in patients who have daily events and a single semiology. Patients with less frequent events or those with multiple semiologies are best served by inpatient video EEG monitoring. Likewise, patients on ASMs should be considered for inpatient video EEG so that medications can be safely withdrawn depending on the clinical context. Each different semiology should be captured to avoid doubt and ensure that there is no concurrent epilepsy.

EMU studies have shown ~10–33% of patients with NEEs have comorbid epilepsy [19–21].

TREATMENT

Delivering the Diagnosis

Proper delivery of diagnosis is the first step in treatment and can be very effective. Around a third of patients can be event free within 6 months after delivery of diagnosis alone [3, 22, 23]. Whenever possible, the diagnosis should be jointly delivered by a neurologist and a mental health provider. The following is an approach to this delivery [24–26]:

(1) If video EEG is used, explain how it works and how this led to the diagnosis.

(2) Express understanding that these are genuine symptoms and you do not think that they are faking.

(3) State the diagnosis of NEEs. Provide other names that the patient may have heard and give reasons as to why those terms are not preferred.

(4) Reassure that this is a common condition.

(5) Talk about predisposing factors such as stress, which can be physical or emotional and can be ongoing or remote. Explain that not everyone has easily identifiable stressors.

(6) Discuss treatment. Explain that ASMs are not effective since they do not have epilepsy.

(7) Explain the treatment is psychological therapy, with CBT being commonly preferred, and you would like to refer them to a psychologist.

(8) Explain that you will continue to follow them in clinic to ensure that they get the proper treatment and monitor improvement.

(9) Discuss expectations. Explain that it is expected that these will get better and can resolve with treatment.

CBT and Medications

Cognitive behavioral therapy (CBT) is the gold-standard treatment for NEEs [27, 28]. It is important that the mental health provider is familiar with NEEs. Ideally, the neurologist should develop a strong working relationship with a psychologist for referral. This can help avoid miscommunications about the diagnosis or doubt on the part of the psychologist. It is also helpful if the treating psychologist is present at the time of diagnosis, though this is often not logistically possible.

Though CBT is the treatment of choice, the addition of an antidepressant may have a modest additional benefit [27]. Note a randomized trial did not indicate an antidepressant alone altered the frequency of NEEs [27]. Treatment with antidepressants should only be in patients with clinical signs and symptoms of depression. Patients with symptoms of depression, anxiety, or other psychiatric conditions likely benefit from referral to a psychiatrist in addition to psychotherapy.

Withdrawal of ASMs for NEE patients

Antiseizure medicines can be safely withdrawn in patients whom all current event types have been captured and determined nonepileptic, if no other features are concerning for concurrent epilepsy [29]. Patients with epilepsy risk factors, past events suspicious of epileptic seizures, history of events in childhood, or abnormal interictal EEG may be at increased risk for uncovering a concurrent epilepsy upon ASM withdrawal [29]. Antiseizure medicines may still be withdrawn in such patients, though individual risk/benefit needs to be determined based on best clinical judgment.

The optimal time for ASM withdrawal may vary depending on the patient and situation. Patients are commonly taken off ASMs as an inpatient during video EEG monitoring. After the diagnosis is made, ASMs that have been paused during video EEG should not be restarted. If ASMs may be providing alternate benefit (i.e., lamotrigine and mood, topiramate and migraines, etc.), continuation for that indication is appropriate. In that situation, it is vital to educate your patient and document the nonepilepsy rationale for remaining on an ASM to prevent diagnostic confusion for outside medical personnel.

In patients whose ASMs have not been stopped for evaluation, a relatively quick taper over 3 weeks to 1 month per ASM can be utilized. Some ASMs, like benzodiazepines or barbiturates, may require longer tapers due to withdrawal symptoms. If a patient is on multiple ASMs, it may be beneficial to have a clinic visit after ASM withdrawal to ensure no new events concerning for epileptic seizures have arisen.

General Psychiatric Care for Epilepsy Patients

Anxiety and depression are very common comorbid conditions in people with epilepsy. A 2017 metaanalysis found a pooled prevalence of anxiety and depressive disorders of 20.2 and 22.9%, respectively, in people with epilepsy [30]. This is about 2–2.5 times the rates in the general population [31, 32].

Comorbid anxiety and depression have been shown to negatively impact patients' quality of life independent of seizure control [33]. Also, the suicide rate among people with epilepsy has been shown to be 22% higher than that of the general population [34]. Despite this, psychiatric comorbidities often go unrecognized and untreated in people with epilepsy [32, 35].

PSYCHIATRIC MANAGEMENT IN EPILEPSY PATIENTS

Consultation with a psychiatrist can be offered to patients who shows signs or symptoms of psychiatric comorbidity. However, due to the high prevalence and subsequent need, it is sometimes difficult to get patients in with psychiatry in a timely manner. It is therefore important to familiarize yourself with routine psychiatric treatment.

Most SSRIs and SNRIs have been shown to be safe in patients with epilepsy [36]. Four antidepressants do show increased incidence of seizures and should be avoided if possible. These include bupropion, clomipramine, amoxapine, and maprotiline [36, 37]. Prior to starting a medication, other causes of psychiatric symptoms should be excluded, such as [38]:

- Ensure symptoms aren't a side effect of a current ASM
- Assess whether symptoms were uncovered after discontinuation of an ASM with anxiolytic or mood-stabilizing properties
- Ensure the symptoms are not directly preictal, ictal, or postictal. Such symptoms do not respond well to antidepressants [39, 40].

The choice of SSRI and SNRI depends on medical comorbidities and drug interactions. Do not start these medications in patients with bipolar disorder as this can precipitate manic episodes [41]. Urgent referral to psychiatry is best in these cases. Other commonly encountered situations to be aware of include:

- Most SSRIs are substrates of the CYP enzyme system, thus must be managed accordingly when taken with ASMs that are CYP inducers or inhibitors [42]
- Many SSRIs inhibit some of the CYP isoenzymes except for citalopram and escitalopram, thus using citalopram or escitalopram may be best when using ASMs that are also CYP substrates [43, 44]
- Both SSRIs and SNRIs can cause hyponatremia from SIADH [45, 46]. They should be used with caution, and check sodium more frequently in patients on carbamazepine, oxcarbazepine, and eslicarbazepine
- Adverse effects that can be worsened when combining SSRIs and SNRIs with some ASMs include weight gain, sexual adverse effects, and osteopenia and osteoporosis [38].

Depressive symptoms in patients with epilepsy may also respond to CBT, thus patients should be offered referrals in addition to medication or alternately, as initial therapy if felt medically safe [47, 48].

ADHD is a commonly encountered psychiatric comorbidity in children with epilepsy [49]. Though not as common in adults, ADHD is likely to be encountered by epilepsy providers. Treatment often involves stimulant medications and its strongly recommended for a psychiatrist to manage such medications. The most recent evidence suggests individual use of ADHD medications slightly lowered the risk of seizures [50]. This contradicts previous literature that suggest that stimulants increase seizure risk [51–54]. Thus, it is reasonable to consider stimulant therapy assuming you undergo an appropriate risk/benefit discussion with your patient.

Works Cited

1. NM Bodde, JL Brooks, GA Baker et al. Psychogenic non-epileptic seizures – definition, etiology, treatment and prognostic issues: A critical review. *Seizure*. 2009;18(8):543–53.

2. SR Benbadis and W Allen Hauser. An estimate of the prevalence of psychogenic non-epileptic seizures. *Seizure*. 2000;9(4):280–1.

3. R Duncan, S Razvi, and S Mulhern. Newly presenting psychogenic nonepileptic seizures: Incidence, population characteristics, and early outcome from a prospective audit of a first seizure clinic. *Epilepsy Behav*. 2011;20(2):308–11.

4. KR Sigurdardottir and E Olafsson. Incidence of psychogenic seizures in adults: A population-based study in Iceland. *Epilepsia*. 1998;39(7):749–52.

5. JP Szaflarski, M Szaflarski, C Hughes et al. Psychopathology and quality of life: Psychogenic non-epileptic seizures versus epilepsy. *Med Sci Monit*. 2003;9(4):Cr113–18.

6. WC LaFrance, Jr. and SR Benbadis. Avoiding the costs of unrecognized psychological nonepileptic seizures. *Neurology*. 2006;66(11):1620–1.

7. SR Benbadis, E O'Neill, WO Tatum, and L Heriaud. Outcome of prolonged video-EEG monitoring at a typical referral epilepsy center. *Epilepsia*. 2004;45(9):1150–3.

8. SG Jones, TJ O'Brien, SJ Adams et al. Clinical characteristics and outcome in patients with psychogenic nonepileptic seizures. *Psychosom Med*. 2010;72(5):487–97.

9. M Reuber, G Fernández, J Bauer, C Helmstaedter, and CE Elger. Diagnostic delay in psychogenic nonepileptic seizures. *Neurology*. 2002;58(3):493–5.

10. WT Kerr, EA Janio, JM Le et al. Diagnostic delay in psychogenic seizures and the association with anti-seizure medication trials. *Seizure*. 2016;40:123–6.

11. A Avbersek and S Sisodiya. Does the primary literature provide support for clinical signs used to distinguish psychogenic nonepileptic seizures from epileptic seizures? *J Neurol Neurosurg Psychiatry*. 2010;81(7):719–25.

12. TU Syed, WC LaFrance, Jr., ES Kahriman et al. Can semiology predict psychogenic nonepileptic seizures? A prospective study. *Ann Neurol*. 2011;69(6):997–1004.

13. NJ Azar, TF Tayah, L Wang, Y Song, and BW Abou-Khalil. Postictal breathing pattern distinguishes epileptic from nonepileptic convulsive seizures. *Epilepsia*. 2008;49(1):132–7.

14. JR Gates, V Ramani, S Whalen, and R Loewenson. Ictal characteristics of pseudoseizures. *Arch Neurol*. 1985;42(12):1183–7.

15. TR Henry and I Drury. Ictal behaviors during nonepileptic seizures differ in patients with temporal lobe interictal epileptiform EEG activity and patients without interictal epileptiform EEG abnormalities. *Epilepsia*. 1998;39(2):175–82.

16. CW Bazil and TS Walczak. Effects of sleep and sleep stage on epileptic and nonepileptic seizures. *Epilepsia*. 1997;38(1):56–62.

17. R Duncan, M Oto, AJ Russell, and P Conway. Pseudosleep events in patients with psychogenic non-epileptic seizures: Prevalence and associations. *J Neurol Neurosurg Psychiatry*. 2004;75(7):1009–12.

18. BJ Davis. Predicting nonepileptic seizures utilizing seizure frequency, EEG, and response to medication. *Eur Neurol*. 2004;51(3):153–6.

19. SR Benbadis, V Agrawal, and WO Tatum. How many patients with psychogenic nonepileptic seizures also have epilepsy? *Neurology*. 2001;57(5):915–17.

20. S Chen-Block, BW Abou-Khalil, A Arain et al. Video-EEG results and clinical characteristics in patients with psychogenic nonepileptic spells: The effect of a coexistent epilepsy. *Epilepsy Behav*. 2016;62:62–5.

21. H El-Naggar, P Moloney, P Widdess-Walsh et al. Simultaneous occurrence of nonepileptic and epileptic seizures during a single period of in-patient video-electroencephalographic monitoring. *Epilepsia Open*. 2017;2(4):467–71.

22. AM Kanner, J Parra, M Frey et al. Psychiatric and neurologic predictors of psychogenic pseudoseizure outcome. *Neurology*. 1999;53(5):933–8.

23. AM Arain, AM Hamadani, S Islam, and BW Abou-Khalil. Predictors of early seizure remission after diagnosis of psychogenic nonepileptic seizures. *Epilepsy Behav*. 2007;11(3):409–12.

24. WC LaFrance, Jr., M Reuber, and LH Goldstein. Management of psychogenic nonepileptic seizures. *Epilepsia*. 2013;54(suppl. 1):53–67.

25. R Duncan. Psychogenic nonepileptic seizures: Diagnosis and initial management. *Expert Rev Neurother*. 2010;10(12):1803–9.

26. L Hall-Patch, R Brown, A House et al. Acceptability and effectiveness of a strategy for the communication of the diagnosis of psychogenic nonepileptic seizures. *Epilepsia*. 2010;51(1):70–8.

27. WC LaFrance, Jr., GL Baird, JJ Barry et al. Multicenter pilot treatment trial for psychogenic nonepileptic seizures: A randomized clinical trial. *JAMA Psychiatry*. 2014;71(9):997–1005.

28. LH Goldstein, EJ Robinson, JDC Mellers et al. Cognitive behavioural therapy for adults with dissociative seizures (CODES): A pragmatic, multicentre, randomised controlled trial. *Lancet Psychiatry*. 2020;7(6):491–505.

29. M Oto, C Espie, A Pelosi, M Selkirk, and R Duncan. The safety of antiepileptic drug withdrawal in patients with non-epileptic seizures. *J Neurol Neurosurg Psychiatry*. 2005;76(12):1682–5.

30. AJ Scott, L Sharpe, C Hunt, and M Gandy. Anxiety and depressive disorders in people with epilepsy: A meta-analysis. *Epilepsia*. 2017;58(6):973–82.

31. RC Kessler, WT Chiu, O Demler, KR Merikangas, and EE Walters. Prevalence, severity, and comorbidity of 12-month DSM-IV disorders in the National Comorbidity Survey Replication. *Arch Gen Psychiatry*. 2005;62(6):617–27.

32. KM Fiest, SB Patten, KC Altura et al. Patterns and frequency of the treatment of depression in persons with epilepsy. *Epilepsy Behav*. 2014;39:59–64.

33. EK Johnson, JE Jones, M Seidenberg, and BP Hermann. The relative impact of anxiety, depression, and clinical seizure features on health-related quality of life in epilepsy. *Epilepsia*. 2004;45(5):544–50.

34. N Tian, W Cui, M Zack et al. Suicide among people with epilepsy: A population-based analysis of data from the U.S. National Violent Death Reporting System, 17 states, 2003–2011. *Epilepsy Behav*. 2016;61:210–17.

35. MF O'Donoghue, DM Goodridge, K Redhead, JW Sander, and JS Duncan. Assessing the psychosocial consequences of epilepsy: A community-based study. *Br J Gen Pract*. 1999;49(440):211–14.

36. K Alper, KA Schwartz, RL Kolts, and A Khan. Seizure incidence in psychopharmacological clinical trials: An analysis of Food and Drug Administration (FDA) summary basis of approval reports. *Biol Psychiatry*. 2007;62(4):345–54.

37. PC Jobe, JW Dailey, and JF Wernicke. A noradrenergic and serotonergic hypothesis of the linkage between epilepsy and affective disorders. *Crit Rev Neurobiol*. 1999;13(4):317–56.

38. AM Kanner. Most antidepressant drugs are safe for patients with epilepsy at therapeutic doses: A review of the evidence. *Epilepsy Behav*. 2016;61:282–6.

39. P Blanchet and GP Frommer. Mood change preceding epileptic seizures. *J Nerv Ment Dis*. 1986;174(8):471–6.

40. AM Kanner, A Soto, and H Gross-Kanner. Prevalence and clinical characteristics of postictal psychiatric symptoms in partial epilepsy. *Neurology*. 2004;62(5):708–13.

41. RMA Hirschfeld, CL Bowden, MJ Gitlin et al. Practice guideline for the treatment of patients with bipolar disorder (revision). *FOCUS*. 2003;1(1):64–110.

42. PN Patsalos and E Perucca. Clinically important drug interactions in epilepsy: Interactions between antiepileptic drugs and other drugs. *Lancet Neurol*. 2003;2(8):473–81.

43. MH Nelson, AK Birnbaum, and RP Remmel. Inhibition of phenytoin hydroxylation in human liver microsomes by several selective serotonin re-uptake inhibitors. *Epilepsy Res*. 2001;44(1):71–82.

44. EM Haney, SJ Warden, and MM Bliziotes. Effects of selective serotonin reuptake inhibitors on bone health in adults: Time for recommendations about screening, prevention and management? *Bone*. 2010;46(1):13–17.

45. S Jacob and SA Spinler. Hyponatremia associated with selective serotonin-reuptake inhibitors in older adults. *Ann Pharmacother*. 2006;40(9):1618–22.

46. C Andrade. Stahl's essential psychopharmacology: Neuroscientific basis and practical applications. *Mens Sana Monogr*. 2010;8(1):146–50.

47. NJ Thompson, ER Walker, N Obolensky et al. Distance delivery of mindfulness-based cognitive therapy for depression: Project UPLIFT. *Epilepsy Behav*. 2010;19(3):247–54.

48. P Ciechanowski, N Chaytor, J Miller et al. PEARLS depression treatment for individuals with epilepsy: A randomized controlled trial. *Epilepsy Behav*. 2010;19(3):225–31.

49. DW Dunn, JK Austin, and SM Perkins. Prevalence of psychopathology in childhood epilepsy: Categorical and dimensional measures. *Dev Med Child Neurol*. 2009;51(5):364–72.

50. KK Wiggs, Z Chang, PD Quinn et al. Attention-deficit/hyperactivity disorder medication and seizures. *Neurology*. 2018;90(13):e1104–10.

51. DJ Feeney and WM Klykylo. Medication-induced seizures. *J Am Acad Child Adolesc Psychiatry*. 1997;36(8):1018–19.

52. M Goetz, CB Surman, E Mlynarova, and P Krsek. Status epilepticus associated with the administration of long-acting methylphenidate in a 7-year-old girl. *J Clin Psychopharmacol*. 2012;32(2):300–2.

53. M Schertz and T Steinberg. Seizures induced by the combination treatment of methylphenidate and sertraline. *J Child Adolesc Psychopharmacol*. 2008;18(3):301–3.

54. SA Tavakoli and OC Gleason. Seizures associated with venlafaxine, methylphenidate, and zolpidem. *Psychosomatics*. 2003;44(3):262–4.

11

What Are Essential Pediatric Epilepsy Clinical Diagnoses and Treatment Plans?

Pediatric epilepsy is an extraordinarily broad topic. The comprehensive coverage of this subject could warrant its own manual. Since that is not feasible within this manual, this chapter seeks to outline several key diagnoses and respective management that are commonly seen. The chapter begins with febrile seizures before progressing to the select epileptic encephalopathies. It then proceeds to discuss self-limited childhood epilepsies and genetic generalized epilepsies. It finally concludes with the two hemispheric epilepsies: hemimegalencephaly (HE) and Rasmussen's encephalitis (RE).

Febrile Seizures

These are seizures that occur only during febrile illness in children in absence of another acute symptomatic etiology (e.g., an intracranial infection, brain trauma, or metabolic disturbances) and without a history of previous afebrile seizures [1]. The definition has evolved over time, mostly by patient age range.

- International League Against Epilepsy (1993): 1 month–5 years old [2]
- National Institutes of Health: 3 months–5 years old [3]
- American Academy of Pediatrics (2008): 6 months–5 years old [1].

EPIDEMIOLOGY, ETIOLOGY, AND PREDISPOSING FACTORS

Incidence: 2–5% in the white population, 8–10% in the Asian population. No sex differences [4].

Age of peak incidence: 18–24 months, with 90% occurring before age 3 years [4].

Etiology: Unknown, although with 20–40% of patients having a family history, a high genetic susceptibility of polygenic inheritance is thought likely [4].

HIGH YIELD ASSOCIATIONS AND PREDISPOSING FACTORS

Genetic Epilepsy with Febrile Seizures Plus

- Characterized by the coexistence in the same family of at least two individuals with febrile seizures or febrile seizures plus.
- *Febrile seizures plus* are defined as febrile seizures beyond age 6 years or the presence of unprovoked afebrile seizures (regardless of the age) in an individual with febrile seizures.
- A broad phenotypical spectrum is reported, with myoclonic atonic epilepsy (MAE) and Dravet syndrome (DS), two of the most severe forms.
- Genetic epilepsy with febrile seizures plus (GEFS+) has been associated with genetic mutations affecting the subunits of voltage-gated sodium channels (SCN1A, SCN2A, and SCN1B) and GABA-A receptor (GABRG2) [5, 6].

Human Herpes Virus (HHV) 6B Infection

- Identified in a third of the cases [7].
- Febrile status epilepticus (SE) is considered a risk factor for development of mesial temporal sclerosis [8].

Other

- Low birth weight, short gestational age, and fetal growth retardation.
- Use of whole-cell diphtheria/tetanus/pertussis and measles vaccine has been associated with febrile seizures, while the newer acellular diphtheria, tetanus and pertussis (DTaP) vaccine has not been [4].

FEBRILE SEIZURES CLASSIFICATION

- *Simple* are the most common type.
  - Last for <15 minutes
  - Are generalized tonic clonic seizures (GTCs)
  - Occur once in a 24-hour period.
- *Complex* account for 20–30% of febrile seizures.
  - Last for >15 minutes
  - May have a focal onset
  - Recur in 24 hours or during the same illness [9].

DIAGNOSIS AND TREATMENT

Acute Management

1. If actively seizing, first assess "ABC" (airway, breathing, circulation).
2. Reduce the fever with antipyretic agents and initiate specific treatment of the source of fever.
3. Antiseizure medicine (ASM) initiation is usually not needed.
   A. To reaffirm, ASMs do not decrease the potential evolution to eventual epilepsy.
4. In the setting of prolonged febrile seizures (>5 minutes) or SE, lorazepam 0.1 mg/kg should be administered.
   A. To reinforce, SE of any kind is a medical emergency.

5. If ASM treatment is needed (complex febrile seizure or febrile SE), keep in mind:
   A. Sodium channel blockers can worsen suspected sodium channelopathies.
   B. Valproate can worsen patients with possible mitochondrial disease.

Diagnostic Work-Up

A superior history and physical remains crucial and typically establishes the diagnosis. These should be focused on identifying the fever focus. It should simultaneously rule out other acute symptomatic seizure etiologies, particularly meningoencephalitis.

Your focused history should specifically establish:

- Symptoms and context (recent activities, sick contacts, daycare attendance)
- Seizure semiology
- Seizure duration and recovery time
- Timing between the seizure
- Perinatal history
- History of prior central nervous system (CNS) insults
- Personal or family history of seizures/epilepsy
- Immunization status
- Recent changes in medications.

No further tests are recommended for a febrile seizure patient if:

- Seizure is self-limited
- A non-CNS fever focus is identified
- There is low suspicion for other concurrent etiologies responsible for the fever and the seizure
- The patient is clinically stable.

If your patient does not fulfill these criteria, the following tests should be considered.

- Lumbar puncture if:
  - There is a presence of meningeal signs (Kernig's or Brudzinski's sign)
  - There are symptoms or a clinical history concerning for an intracranial infection
  - Receiving prior antibiotic treatment (optional)
  - They are an infant between 6 and 12 months old who are not immunized against *Haemophilus influenzae* type B or *Streptococcus pneumoniae* or their immunization status is unknown (optional) [10].
- Neuroimaging (computerized tomography [CT] and/or magnetic resonance imaging [MRI]) is not recommended unless there is a concern for an acute neurological condition other than the febrile seizure, such as a presence of focal neurological symptoms or if there is febrile SE [4].
- Electroencephalogram (EEG)
  - Not recommended in neurologically healthy patients with a simple febrile seizure [10].
  - It is recommended for prolonged febrile seizures or SE.
  - Focal EEG slowing or attenuation suggests acute neuronal injury with potential long-term consequences [11].
- Lab tests are not required after a simple febrile seizure [10].
  - Labs should be obtained if suspicion for metabolic derangements or coagulopathy. Other diagnostic studies may be indicated (i.e., urinalysis, blood culture, etc.) if the source of fever is unclear.

LONG-TERM MANAGEMENT AFTER FIRST FEBRILE SEIZURE

Fevers should be aggressively managed with antipyretic treatment as soon as the fever is identified, although the risk of febrile seizure or seizure recurrence is not lessened. Identification and treatment of the source of fever is crucial each time. Routine genetic testing is not recommended unless you have clear suspicion for GEFS+ or DS.

PROGNOSIS FOR PATIENTS WITH FEBRILE SEIZURES

A third of patients may have recurrent febrile seizures [4]. Younger age at first febrile seizure increases the risk of recurrence. For instance, 50% of patients under 1 year may have recurrent febrile seizures, while only 20% of patients over 3 years have recurrent febrile seizures [12]. Other risk factors for recurrent febrile seizures include:

1. Low-grade fever at the time of seizure presentation
2. A short interval between fever onset and seizure occurrence
3. A history of febrile seizures in a first-degree relative.

The duration of the first febrile seizure or febrile seizure type (simple versus complex) is not associated with febrile seizures recurrence risk [12]. However, prolonged first febrile seizures are associated with recurrent prolonged febrile seizures [4]. The risk of epilepsy for febrile seizure patients is 2–5%, higher than the 1–2% in the general population. The main risk factors for progression from febrile seizure to subsequent epilepsy include [9, 13]:

1. A history of developmental delay
2. An abnormal focal neurological exam prior to the febrile seizures
3. A complex febrile seizure, which includes febrile SE
4. A history of epilepsy in a first-degree relative
5. Four or more febrile seizures
6. Age at onset of >3 years.

You should counsel that simple febrile seizures have not been associated with adverse neuropsychological development. However, data are less clear for patients with prolonged febrile seizures or febrile SE.

Developmental and Epileptic Encephalopathies

Developmental encephalopathies are characterized by impairment related to etiologies independent of epilepsy. In contrast, epileptic encephalopathies refer to specific epilepsy diagnoses that worsen developmental decline separate from the underlying developmental etiology alone [14]. The most common epileptic encephalopathies will be discussed in this chapter, excluding early infantile encephalopathies.

INFANTILE SPASMS SYNDROME

Epileptic spasms require urgent evaluation for diagnosis and management. They are semiologically defined as brief tonic (flexor, extensor, or mixed) contractions of axial muscles. This can be symmetric or asymmetric. They commonly last <3 seconds. Infantile spasms tend to occur in clusters and are seen frequently on awakening.

Patients with the classic West syndrome (triad of epileptic spasms, hypsarrhythmia on EEG, and developmental regression) and infants without West syndrome can have infantile spasms [15].

Etiology: Numerous etiologies can cause infantile spasms syndrome (ISS), whether congenital or acquired. A genetic cause is identified in ≥41% of cases [16]. Careful neurological and general exam (specifically dermatologic and ophthalmologic) are essential to establish an underlying cause.

Clinical picture: They typically start around 3–12 months, although can range from 1–24 months. Developmental arrest or regression can precede or coincide with epileptic spasm onset. When focal seizures occur, a structural brain abnormality should be assessed. Infantile spasms syndrome typically evolves to drug-resistant epilepsy (DRE), particularly Lennox–Gastaut syndrome (LGS).

EEG: The classic interictal finding is *hypsarrhythmia* (disorganized high amplitude excessive slowing with multifocal epileptiform discharges). Some infants have abundant multifocal epileptiform discharges without the chaotic background seen in hypsarrhythmia. The ictal pattern is a high-amplitude generalized sharp or slow wave followed by low-amplitude fast activity (also termed electrodecrement).

MRI is abnormal in one half to two-thirds of patients.

ISS management: The first step is urgent/emergent treatment initiation with adrenocorticotropic hormone (ACTH). Prednisone and vigabatrin are second-line agents. One key exception is in tuberous sclerosis with epileptic spasms, where vigabatrin is the treatment of choice. In addition, a trial of pyridoxine 100 mg/day for 3–7 days should be considered if no etiology is found and pyridoxine-dependent epilepsy cannot be ruled out [15].

Prompt evaluation with MRI should be performed. It should be repeated after 2 years of age once myelination is complete if no other etiologies are found. Genetic and metabolic studies are frequently sought, particularly if there is no causative MRI lesion found.

DRAVET SYNDROME

Etiology: A pathogenic variant of SCN1A has been found in nearly 80% of cases. Rare mutations in the GABRG2, GABRA1, STXBP1, and SCN1B genes have also been described. The etiology of about 20% of DS patients remains unknown.

Clinical picture: This diagnosis should be strongly considered in a normally developing child who presents with prolonged febrile and afebrile seizures (typically hemiclonic), between 3 and 9 months of age. Epileptic spasms exclude a DS diagnosis and rather suggest ISS. Additional seizure types (myoclonic, atypical absences, etc.) and progressive developmental slowing follows soon after between the age of 1 and 4 years [15].

Behavioral disorders are frequently comorbid. Gait abnormalities and mild pyramidal signs may be noted starting in late childhood. Frequent seizures and SE are not uncommon before the age of 5 years. These decrease in frequency by adolescence/early adulthood.

EEG: Studies obtained prior to 2 years of age can be normal or may show background slowing. Diffuse slowing with multifocal and generalized epileptiform discharges begin after 2 year of age.

MRI: Similar to EEG, they can be normal at seizure onset. Mild cerebral and cerebellar atrophy may appear over time. A third of the patients will develop hippocampal sclerosis.

DS treatment: Given the sodium channel (SCN1A) mutation, use of sodium channel–blocking drugs like phenytoin, carbamazepine and derivates, and lamotrigine characteristically worsen seizures in DS and should be avoided.

Cannabidiol has been approved as adjunctive therapy [17].

Stiripentol has been approved as an adjuvant treatment for patients with DS who are also taking clobazam and are 2 years of age and older [18].

Fenfluramine has been approved for patients with DS age 2 years and older. It can be used as adjunctive treatment in patients receiving stiripentol [19]. Monitoring for valvular heart disease and pulmonary hypertension is mandatory.

GLUCOSE TRANSPORTER TYPE 1 DEFICIENCY SYNDROME

Etiology: Caused by pathogenic variant mutations of the SLC2A1 gene, which codes for glucose transporter type 1 (Glut1). This causes impaired glucose transport across the blood–brain barrier. This informs the treatment described.

Clinical picture: This diagnosis presents with multiple neurological symptoms. It should be suspected for infants or children presenting with seizures that are particularly triggered with fasting. Other neurological symptoms include movement disorders like dystonia as well as cognitive delay or regression. Seizures are those of generalized semiology including myoclonic, GTC, atonic, or atypical absences. Focal semiologies are rare. There may be microcephaly (in 50% of the cases) or deceleration of head growth [15].

EEG: Although sometimes initially normal, generalized 2.5–4 Hz spike and wave are seen in children older than 2 years of age.

MRI: Nonspecific abnormalities such as hyperintensity of subcortical U-fibers, prominence of perivascular Virchow spaces, prominent ventricles, and delayed myelination for age manifest in 25% of patients.

Labs: Given impaired glucose transport, low CSF glucose or lactate with normal blood glucose after 4–6 hours of fasting are indicative. A lumbar puncture may be omitted if phenotype is compatible and of course if genetic testing is positive for a pathogenic variant. If clinical suspicion remains in the setting of normal lumbar puncture and genetic testing, consider erythrocyte-uptake testing and the measurement of Glut1 on the surface of red blood cells.

Management: The ketogenic diet is first-line treatment. Essentially, the brain uses ketones as an alternate fuel source since glucose is unable to be efficiently transported across the blood–brain barrier [20].

MYOCLONIC ATONIC EPILEPSY

This was previously known by the eponym Doose syndrome.

Etiology: Unlike the previous diagnoses, MAE has a complex polygenic inheritance. Pathogenic variants in the following genes have been reported: SCN1A, SCN1B, SCN2A, STX1B, SLC6A1, CHD2, SYNGAP1, NEXMIF, and KIAA2022. Pathogenic variants of SLC2A1 have been noted in 5% of patients with MAE.

Clinical picture: This presents with an abrupt onset of seizures at around the age of 2–6 years, affecting boys more than girls. Not unexpectedly, myoclonic atonic semiology must be present for the diagnosis. Still, myoclonic, atonic, absence, and GTCs can also be seen. Nonconvulsive SE may be the form of presentation. Epileptic spasms and focal seizures exclude an MAE diagnosis [14].

Development is normal for two-thirds of children prior to seizure onset. After that, developmental plateauing or regression may occur. Similar to other epileptic encephalopathies, behavioral disturbances are commonly comorbid.

Seizures are typically drug resistant initially. In a less common note of positivity for epileptic encephalopathies, two-thirds of children achieve remission within 3 years of onset and developmental progress is noted. The remaining third may experience seizure persistence, cognitive impairment, aggression, and hyperactivity.

EEG: This may be normal at onset. Monomorphic biparietal theta rhythms are characteristic but do not occur in all patients. As the disease progresses, there is background slowing with generalized 3–6 Hz spike and slow wave or polyspike and slow wave. The ictal pattern for myoclonic atonic seizures shows a generalized polyspike or spike with the myoclonus, followed by a high-voltage slow wave associated with the atonic component.

MRI is normal for children with MAE.

Management: Sodium channel blockers (carbamazepine, lamotrigine, phenytoin, etc.) should be avoided. Broad-spectrum ASMs are the mainstay. The ketogenic diet may also be considered.

LENNOX–GASTAUT SYNDROME

Etiology: This diagnosis represents the evolution from a previous severe infantile epilepsy or syndrome. Patients with ISS comprise 20% of LGS patients.

Clinical picture: The classic clinical scenario is a child with [14]:

1. Multiple seizures types (must have tonic seizures)
    A. Apart from tonic seizures, at least one other seizure type is mandatory
        i.   Absence seizures
        ii. Atonic seizures
        iii. Myoclonic seizures
        iv. Focal seizures of varying semiology
        v.   GTCs.
2. Generalized slow spike and slow wave complexes ($\leq$2.5 Hz) and generalized paroxysmal fast activity
3. Starting at 3–5 years of age (a range of 18 months–8 years)
4. Accompanying cognitive and behavioral impairment [14].

As children age into adulthood, LGS persists as DRE.

EEG: The background is slow, two interictal patterns are required for the diagnosis [14]

1. Generalized slow spike wave complexes at $\leq$2.5 Hz. It can be abundant and occurring in runs without definite clinical changes
2. Generalized paroxysmal fast activity: bursts of diffuse fast (>10 Hz) activity.

Focal or multifocal epileptiform discharges can be seen. The ictal pattern for tonic seizures shows bilateral >10 Hz with an initial diffuse electrodecrement followed by gradual increase in amplitude.

MRI: Although it can be normal, a structural lesion is identified in most cases.

Labs: Metabolic testing is recommended if no imaging or genetic etiology is identified.

Management: Most ASMs may be considered. More recently, cannabidiol has been approved as an adjunctive treatment consideration [21]. Consider corpus callosotomy specifically for atonic seizures while focal surgery can be palliatively considered if a target is identifiable.

DEVELOPMENTAL AND/OR EPILEPTIC ENCEPHALOPATHY WITH SPIKE AND WAVE ACTIVATION IN SLEEP

There is a spectrum of conditions characterized by dramatic spike wave activation during sleep. It includes the formerly known Landau–Kleffner syndrome, epileptic encephalopathy with continuous spike wave in sleep, and atypical benign partial epilepsy.

Etiology: This is not completely understood, while some are genetic, whether monogenic or complex inheritance.

Clinical picture: While peaking at age 4–5 years, it can occur from ages 2–12 years. Developmental and behavioral regression are the key symptoms with the EEG findings providing the diagnosis [14].

Around puberty, there is tendency toward remission of the seizures and resolution of the epileptic encephalopathy with spike and wave activation in sleep (ESES) activation in sleep. Neurocognitive and behavioral improvement routinely follow, although residual impairment may be seen. Worse neurocognitive outcome is associated with younger age at onset of the syndrome and longer disease duration. Etiology accordingly impacts prognosis.

EEG: Studies are often normal during wakefulness and can alternately show focal or diffuse slowing with intermixed epileptiform discharges. During drowsiness and sleep, almost continuous slow spike and wave in slow sleep are seen. While also seen in stage II sleep, the slow spike/waves tend to decrease or disappear during deeper sleep.

MRI: There is no classic lesion with ESES, as imaging can be lesional or normal.

FEBRILE INFECTION-RELATED EPILEPSY SYNDROME

Etiology: While still hotly debated, febrile infection-related epilepsy syndrome (FIRES) is thought to be a fulminant neuroinflammatory process.

Clinical picture: This entity is defined by its explosive onset as superrefractory SE in a normal developing child (mean age 8 years). A prior febrile infection that started between 2 weeks and 24 hours before is the key temporal association. The acute phase may last 1-12 weeks and carries significant morbidity and mortality. The chronic phase, during which there is often drug-resistant multifocal epilepsy, has concomitant variable cognitive impairment and behavioral disturbances [14].

EEG: The interictal pattern is background slowing with multifocal epileptiform findings. Extreme delta brush can be seen in the frontal and central regions. As implied by superrefractory SE, frequent seizures are sadly the norm.

MRI: This is frustratingly normal in the acute phase in two-thirds of cases, although nonspecific findings of SE may also be. Imaging in the chronic phase reveals diffuse and/or focal atrophy.

Labs: Lumbar puncture is mandatory in order to rule out CNS infection. Mild pleocytosis may be seen. Autoimmune panel and metabolic studies are normal.

Management: A diagnosis of exclusion, FIRES requires ruling out known infectious, metabolic, toxic, and structural etiologies in the first 24-48 hours.

Treatment requires escalating ASM therapies with treatment and sedation according to SE protocols. Avoid prolonged anesthetics since longer duration of barbiturate induced and burst suppression coma have been associated with worse cognitive outcomes.

Consider intravenous methylprednisolone +/- intravenous immunoglobulins (IViGs) after the first 48 hours if autoimmune encephalitis is suspected. If no response by day 6, start the ketogenic diet, consider anakinra (IL-1 receptor antagonist), and cannabidiol. If no response, escalating immunotherapies such as tocilizumab or canakinumab may be considered [22].

Self-Limited Focal Epilepsies of Childhood

This is a group of syndromes that account for 10–20% of all pediatric epilepsies. They represent a functional derangement in the maturing brain, with an inherent excitability of specific brain areas in each syndrome. The brain regions affected inform the characteristic clinical symptoms for each syndrome [23].

Formerly known as "benign focal epilepsies of childhood," the nomenclature was updated by the International League Against Epilepsy in 2017 to reaffirm the tendency for spontaneous remission, but also to highlight the possibility of associated, although rare, neurological comorbidities [24].

Characterized by normal neuroimaging and neurological status, these diagnoses tend to self-resolve prior to adolescence. They may not require ASMs due to low seizure frequency, and specific syndromes have characteristic EEG epileptiform discharges with consistent morphology and location, usually sleep potentiated with a normal background [25]. The main defining features of the four syndromes are characterized in Table 11.1 [14, 23].

An example of centrotemporal benign spikes also known as benign focal epileptiform discharges of childhood (BFEDs), typically seen in SeLECTS (self-limited epilepsy with centrotemporal spikes (formerly known as benign Rolandic epilepsy) is shown in Fig. 11.1. An example of the fixation-off sensitivity phenomenon, which can be seen in certain types of self-limited focal epilepsies of childhood is shown in Fig. 11.2.

Table 11.1 Main features of the different self-limited focal epilepsies of childhood syndromes

	SeLAS	SeLECTS	COVE	POLE
Peak age (years)	3–6	7	8–9	11
Semiology	Initial autonomic symptoms, often emesis Can progress to tonic eye/head deviation followed by hemiclonic or bilateral tonic clonic semiology	Unilateral sensory and motor (tonic or clonic) semiology involving lower face, mouth, or tongue Aphasia or dysarthria Sialorrhea May progress to hemi clonic or bilateral tonic clonic	Visual auras with simple hallucinations Can be associated with ipsilateral eye or head deviation Not triggered by photic stimuli May progress to hemisensory, hemiclonic, or bilateral tonic clonic	Visual auras with simple visual hallucinations Triggered by photic stimuli Ipsilateral eye or head deviation May evolve to bilateral tonic clonic seizure
Seizure frequency and duration	Rare Can be >5 min 50% SE	Rare 1–3 min 5% SE	Frequent 1–3 min	Rare 1–3 min

Table 11.1 (cont.)

	SeLAS	SeLECTS	COVE	POLE
State at seizure onset	Sleep	Sleep	Awake	Awake
Characteristic EEG features	Posteriorly predominant Spikes/SW At times generalized Fixation-off sensitivity phenomenon	Centrotemporal spikes/SW with a transverse dipole (frontal positivity, temporoparietal negativity)	Occipital spikes/SW Fixation-off sensitivity phenomenon	Occipital spikes/ polyspikes facilitated by IPS Fixation-off sensitivity phenomenon

COVE: childhood onset visual epilepsy (formerly known as idiopathic childhood occipital epilepsy Gastaut type); IPS: intermittent photic stimulation; POLE: photosensitive occipital lobe epilepsy (formerly known as idiopathic photosensitive occipital lobe epilepsy); SeLAS: self-limited epilepsy with autonomic seizures (formerly known as Panayiotopoulos syndrome); SW: sharp waves.

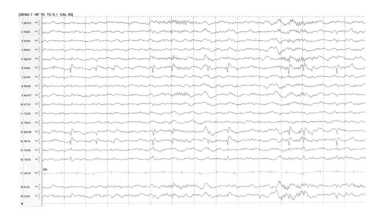

Fig. 11.1 Right centrotemporal BFEDs. Electroencephalogram of a 13-year-old female with a history of two generalized convulsive seizures at the age of 7 and 8 years old, respectively. Note right centrotemporal spikes, forming a horizontal dipole with maximum negativity at C4-T4 and positivity at Fp2-F4 occurring in runs during sleep N2. Potentiation with sleep is a characteristic of BFEDs.

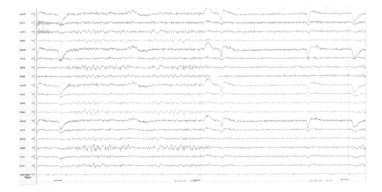

Fig. 11.2 Fixation-off sensitivity phenomenon. This phenomenon refers to the appearance of posterior or generalized epileptiform discharges after removal of visual fixation, such as when using Frenzel glasses or during eye closure. The epileptiform discharges continue as long as the eyes are closed.

Genetic Generalized Epilepsies

IDIOPATHIC GENERALIZED EPILEPSIES

These diagnoses are group of syndromes of presumed genetic (mainly polygenic) etiology. They are characterized by [26]:

1. The presence of one or the combination of the following generalized seizure types. Each seizure type is predominant depending on the syndrome.
   a. Absence
   b. Myoclonic
   c. Tonic clonic
   d. Myoclonic tonic clonic
   e. The presence of generalized tonic, atonic, myoclonic atonic, epileptic spasms, or focal seizures excludes an idiopathic generalized epilepsy (IGE) diagnosis.
2. Particular range of age at onset for each syndrome.
3. Characteristic generalized spike and slow wave (Fig. 11.3) or polyspikes discharges at 2.5–5.5 Hz on EEG (Fig. 11.4).

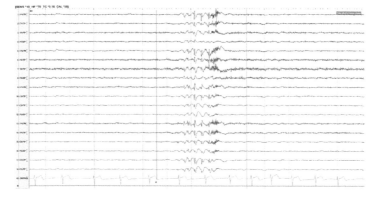

Fig. 11.3 Generalized spike and slow wave complexes at 3 Hz. 26-year-old male with past medical history of juvenile myoclonic epilepsy.

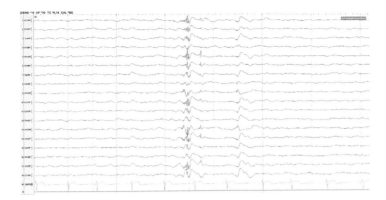

Fig. 11.4 Generalized polyspikes. Same patient as Fig. 11.3.

    a. Generalized spike wave may appear fragmented and not consistently in one location.

4. No association with intellectual impairment, although learning disorder or attention deficit disorder may be seen.

5. Good response to broad-spectrum ASMs.

    There may be overlap among syndromes and at times one of them results from the evolution of another IGE syndrome. Table 11.2 highlights the main differences among them [26].

OTHER CHILDHOOD GENETIC GENERALIZED EPILEPSY SYNDROMES

Epilepsy with Myoclonic Absence (Formerly Known as Tassinari Syndrome)

• Peak age at onset: 7 years old, male predominant.

Predominant seizure type: Myoclonic absence seizures are characterized by absence seizures accompanied by tonic abduction of the arms with superimposed rhythmic 3 Hz jerks. Generalized tonic

Table 11.2 Main features of the different IGE syndromes

	CAE	JAE	JME	GTCA
Peak age at onset in years (range)	4–10 (2–13)	9–13 (8–20)	10–24 (8–40)	10–25 (5–40)
Predominant seizure type	Absence	Absence, less frequent than CAE	Myoclonic	Only GTC
Seizure triggers	Hyperventilation	Hyperventilation	Sleep deprivation Photic stimulation	Sleep deprivation
Interictal EEG	2.5–4 Hz GSWC OIRDA in 30%	3–5.5 Hz GSWC	3–5.5 Hz GSWC or polyspikes	3–5.5 Hz GSWC
Treatment considerations	ETX first line	ETX in monotherapy not recommended due to presence of GTCS	Valproate is most effective, although avoid in women of child bearing age Lamotrigine may worsen myoclonus in some patients	Valproate, avoid in women of child-bearing age Lamotrigine and levetiracetam are also reasonable options as a first choice Add on perampanel in pharmacoresistant cases

Prognosis	60% remit by adolescence, remaining may evolve to other IGE syndromes	Drug responsive but lifelong	Drug responsive but lifelong	Drug responsive but lifelong
Other considerations	If onset before age 4 or atypical features, consider genetic testing and evaluation for Glut1 deficiency syndrome. If prominent myoclonus during an absence, consider E-MA	If independent myoclonus, consider JME. If prominent myoclonus during an absence, consider E-MA	If myoclonic seizures start before age 3 years, consider infantile myoclonic epilepsy	If other seizures types are present, exclude this syndrome

CAE: childhood absence epilepsy; E-MA: epilepsy with myoclonic absences; ETX: ethosuximide; GSWC: generalized spike and slow wave complexes; GTCA: epilepsy with generalized tonic clonic seizures alone; IAE: juvenile absence epilepsy; JME: juvenile myoclonic epilepsy; OIRDA: occipital intermittent rhythmic delta activity clonic seizures, atonic, typical, or atypical absence seizures may also occur [16].

- Seizure triggers: hyperventilation.
- Interictal EEG: 3 Hz spike and slow wave complexes.
- Prognosis: Remission occurs in 40% of the cases. Intellectual disability may be present at onset and may affect up to 70% of the patients overtime. The presence of multiple seizure types is associated with poorer prognosis.

Epilepsy with Eyelid Myoclonia (Formerly Known as Jeavons Syndrome)

- Peak age at onset: 6–8 years old, female predominant.
- Predominant seizure type: Eyelid myoclonus is characterized by 3–6 Hz myoclonic jerks of the eyelids. There is upward gaze deviation and extension of the head with many. Absence seizures can cooccur. Focal seizures exclude the diagnosis [14].
- Seizure triggers: Eye closure and photic stimulation are the main two. "Sun flower syndrome" can be a diagnostic clue as patients can exhibit prominent photic induction and have sun-seeking behavior [14].
- Prognosis: While a lifelong epilepsy, patients respond well to ASMs. Intellectual disability may be seen, particularly in those susceptible to photic stimulation.

NEUROCUTANEOUS SYNDROMES AND EPILEPSY

Neurocutaneous syndromes, also known as phakomatoses, are a heterogenous group of congenital disorders characterized by predilection for neuroectodermal-derived structures such as the brain and the skin. They are frequently multiorgan diseases and benefit from a multidisciplinary approach [25].

The most common neurocutaneous syndromes' features are listed in Table 11.3 [25, 27, 28]. Other neurocutaneous syndromes not covered in

Table 11.3 Most common neurocutaneous syndromes' features

	Tuberous sclerosis	Sturge–Weber	Neurofibromatosis type 1
Genes	TSC 1 gene (CR. 9q34) TSC 2 gene (CR16p13.3) 15% of patients that meet diagnostic criteria do not have pathogenic variant or deletions	GNAQ	NF1 (CR 17 q11.2)
Inheritance	AD Variable expression 60% de novo Consider mosaicism if no pathogenic variant or deletions are detected	Not inherited Occurs from somatic mosaicism from postzygotic mutations	AD Complete penetrance Variable expression Segmental NF is due to somatic mosaicism from postzygotic mutations
Pathogenesis	TSC 1 codes for hamartin TSC 2 codes for tuberin Pathogenic variants activate the mTOR pathway, this causes increased tissue growth and proliferation TSC 1 has a less severe phenotypic expression	GNAQ codes for a subunit of a G protein involved in blood vessel formation Mutation results in angiomatosis Leptomeningeal angioma may produce hypoxic-ischemic injury to adjacent tissue	NF1 codes for neurofibromin NF1 acts as a tumor-suppressor gene NF1 mutations produce a loss of or reduced function

Table 11.3 (cont.)

	Tuberous sclerosis	Sturge–Weber	Neurofibromatosis type 1
Brain lesions	Cortical tubers (Fig. 11.5) White matter lesions Subependymal nodules SEGA	Leptomeningeal angioma (PWS) Choroid plexus hypertrophy	Optic nerve gliomas Low-grade glioma Brainstem gliomas Megalencephaly Cerebrovascular dysplasia
Epilepsy features	80% of patients have epilepsy 70% develop by age 1 Epileptic spasms and focal onset seizures with GTC seizures later in life Can result in LGS EEG findings may correlate with a larger tuber EEG findings may vary overtime	In up to 80% of patients Typically present by age 2 Focal onset motor seizures most frequent type	Epilepsy in 3–6.5% of patients Variable seizure types
Other neurological or psychiatric manifestations	Intellectual disability, particularly associated with early onset seizures Autism Behavioral disturbances Hydrocephalus if obstructive SEGA	Intellectual disability Stroke-like episodes Progressive hemiparesis Homonymous hemianopia Migraine-like headaches	Intellectual disability

Cutaneous stigmata	Hypomelanotic macules (Ash leaf spots) Facial angiofibromas Forehead plaques Shagreen patches Subungueal fibromas	Unilateral facial capillary angioma following V nerve (V1 more frequent) Hemiatrophy	Hyperpigmented (café-au-lait) macules Freckling in intertriginous areas Neurofibromas (can become malignant)
Systemic involvement	Cardiac rhabdomyomas Retinal astrocytomas Angiomyolipomas Dental pits Hepatic cysts Pulmonary lymphangioleiomyomatosis	Choroidal hemangiomas Glaucoma GH deficiency Central hypothyroidism	Lisch nodules Rhabdomyosarcoma GISTs Bone abnormalities Pheochromocytoma Breast cancer
Epilepsy management	VGB ACTH Everolimus (adjunct) Other ASMs and epilepsy surgery following general principles of epilepsy treatment	ASMs and epilepsy surgery following general principles of epilepsy treatment	ASMs and epilepsy surgery following general principles of epilepsy treatment

Table 11.3 (cont.)

	Tuberous sclerosis	Sturge–Weber	Neurofibromatosis type 1
Other management considerations	Brain MRI recommended every 1–3 years to detect SEGA in patients <25 years Periodic renal MRI Periodic blood pressure and GFR assessment Periodic EKG Periodic echocardiogram if cardiac rhabdomyoma Periodic chest HRCT if high risk for lymphangioleiomyomatosis Ophthalmology assessment	Aspirin 3–5 mg/kg/day to prevent hypoxic-ischemic injury Ophthalmology assessment Laser for PWS	Monitor for low growth and precocious puberty Ophthalmology assessment

AD: autosomal dominant; CR: chromosome; EKG: electrocardiogram; GFR: glomerular filtration rate; GH: growth hormone; GIST: gastrointestinal stromal tumor; GNAQ: G protein subunit alpha Q; HRCT: high-resolution CT; mTOR: mammalian target of rapamycin; NF: neurofibromatosis; PWS: Port wine stain; TSC: tuberous sclerosis; SEGA: subependymal giant astrocytoma; VGB: vigabatrin

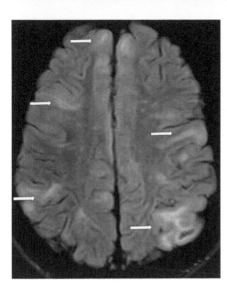

Fig. 11.5 Cortical and subcortical tubers. An axial image from a fluid-attenuated inversion recovery (FLAIR) sequence. Note hyperintensities, prominently in the left parietal lobe, in a patient with tuberous sclerosis and epilepsy.

Table 11.3 but associated with epilepsy are epidermal nevus syndrome, incontinentia pigmenti, hypomelanosis of Ito, and neurocutaneous melanosis [25].

HE and RE

HEMIGMEGALOENCEPHALY

A large malformation of cortical development due to an abnormal, nonneoplastic, cell proliferation resulting in an enlarged and dysplastic hemisphere. It can involve the entire hemisphere or just part of it. Radiological studies have shown the contralateral hemisphere to be smaller compared to nonhemigmegaloencephaly (HE) age-matched controls [29, 30].

- Etiology: Postzygotic mutations result in activation of the phosphatidylinositol 3-kinase (PI3K)/Akt/mammalian target of rapamycin (mTOR) signaling pathways. These mutations abnormally affect pathways crucial for cell survival, growth, and proliferation [25].

- Clinical picture: Focal DRE begins in the neonatal period or early infancy with developmental delay or focal neurological signs appropriate for the dysplastic cortex.
  - Ohtahara syndrome or West syndrome can be a presenting syndrome.
  - Can occur in isolation or in association with neurocutaneous syndromes.
- MRI: Dramatic hemispheric enlargement, at times more focal over frontal or temporoparietal regions (quadrantic dysplasia). Cortex is diffusely abnormal with areas of thickening or thinning and abnormal underlying white matter. Ventricles are typically enlarged and/or distorted. Gray matter heterotopia can be seen.
- Treatment: ASMs have little efficacy. Early anatomical or functional hemispherectomy may improve seizure control and cognition [31].

RASMUSSEN'S ENCEPHALITIS

This is an acquired, progressive, inflammatory disease characterized by unilateral hemispheric atrophy resulting in hemiparesis, DRE, and cognitive decline.

Diagnosis is made by fulfilling agreed upon clinical, EEG, MRI, or histopathological diagnostic criteria [32]. Part A criteria requires all three clinical, EEG, or MRI criteria. Part B criteria can rely on two of three clinical, MRI, or histopathological criteria.

Part A criteria for RE (all 3 required)

Clinical	Focal seizures
	Unilateral cortical deficits
EEG	Unihemispheric slowing with or without epileptiform activity
	Unilateral seizure onset
MRI	Unihemisheric focal cortical atrophy with either:
	1. Gray or white matter T2/FLAIR hyperintense signal
	2. Hyperintense signal or atrophy of the ipsilateral caudate head

Part B criteria for RE (2 of 3 required)

Clinical	Epilepsia partialis continua (EPC)
	or
	Progressive unilateral cortical deficit
MRI	Progressive unihemispheric focal cortical atrophy
	Without a biopsy specimen, MRI with gadolinium and cranial CT should assure the absence of enhancement and calcifications
Histopathology	T cell–predominant encephalitis with activated microglial cells and reactive astrogliosis
	Numerous parenchymal macrophages, B cells, plasma cells, or viral inclusion bodies exclude an RE diagnosis

Epidemiology: A German study showed an annual incidence of 2.4 cases per 10 million aged 18 years and younger [33]. Peak age of onset is 1–13 years with a median of age 6. Still, 10% of cases begin in adolescence or later. There is no predominance by gender, geography, or ethnicity [34].

Etiology and histopathology: The cause of RE is unknown. Histopathological studies show evidence of an immune mediated disease, thought to be cytotoxic CD8+ T cells mediated with additional facilitation by microglia and astroglia. However, the presumed precipitating antigen is unknown.

Focal cortical dysplasia (FCD) or tuberous sclerosis have also been found on series of surgical specimens [35, 36]. This finding, coupled with inflammation associated with FCD type IIb may so preliminarily suggest RE could result from progressive inflammation around an FCD [34].

Three Clinical Phases

1. Prodromal stage: Rasmussen's encephalitis begins as relatively infrequent focal seizures and rare neurological decline. This lasts a mean duration of 7.1 months, ranging from 0 to 8.1 years. Some patients lack a prodromal stage.

2. Acute stage: This stage is characterized by cerebral hemiatrophy, frequent focal seizures, cognitive decline, and progressive focal neurological deficits (hemiparesis, hemianopia, and dysphasia if RE

affects the dominant hemisphere). This phase has a median duration of 8 months (ranging from 4 to 8 months).

3. Residual stage: The last RE stage has persistent, stable neurological and cognitive deficit. Seizure frequency is decreased in comparison to the acute stage.

Epilepsy features: Seizures are expectedly focal at onset with possible evolution to bilateral tonic clonic seizures. Focal motor semiology is most consistently reported, particularly in the form of EPC, occurring in 50% of the patients. Other semiology types such as somatosensory, auditory, and visual auras, among others, have been described and suggest a progression of the disease toward posterior cortical areas.

The EEG shows nonspecific findings and may evolve with time. Background slowing with asymmetric involvement heralds the onset of the disease. The EEG may progress into frequent bilateral epileptiform discharges and seizures that are significantly prominent on the diseased hemisphere. Of note, clinical manifestations of EPC may not be accompanied by an electrographic seizure pattern, so clinical vigilance is key.

Differential diagnosis: As RE is a unilateral disease, considerations should also include unilateral progressive disorders of infectious or autoimmune encephalitis, vasculitis, mitochondrial diseases, Sturge–Weber syndrome, hemiconvulsion-hemiplegia-epilepsy syndrome, and Parry–Romberg syndrome, among others.

Treatment

Antiseizure medicines: RE is characterized by DRE so ASMs have shown limited efficacy.

Immunotherapy: Long-term corticosteroids, IViGs, plasmapheresis, and T cell–inactivating drugs (i.e., tacrolimus and azathioprine) have shown positive results against functional decline and structural damage, without evidence of superiority among them. However, these have proven to be ineffective for epilepsy treatment and prevention of cognitive decline [34].

Surgery: Anatomical hemispherectomy, functional hemispherotomy hemidecortication, and hemispherotomy are the only curative treatment for epilepsy in RE. Hemispherectomy has shown >70% seizure-freedom rates [37]. However, this curative treatment is balanced by expected deficits of contralateral spastic hemiplegia (although preserved ability to walk with rehabilitation), hemianopia, and aphasia with disconnection of the dominant hemisphere.

Given the risk/benefit balance of surgery, timing of surgery is not well established. Some advocate for early surgical intervention as a means of protecting the initially normal contralateral hemisphere and ideally minimizing progressive neurocognitive decline. There is controversy regarding the effect of the disease itself, the age at onset, and age of hemispherectomy/hemispherotomy on language reorganization. In sum, time of surgery should be individualized to the patient after a full discussion and agreement with the patient and family [32, 34].

Works Cited

1. Steering Committee on Quality I, Management SoFSAAoP. Febrile seizures: Clinical practice guideline for the long-term management of the child with simple febrile seizures. *Pediatrics*. 2008;121(6):1281–6.

2. Guidelines for epidemiologic studies on epilepsy. Commission on Epidemiology and Prognosis, International League Against Epilepsy. *Epilepsia*. 1993;34(4):592–6.

3. JM Freeman. Febrile seizures: A consensus of their significance, evaluation, and treatment. *Pediatrics*. 1980;66(6):1009.

4. A Gupta. Febrile seizures. *Continuum (Minneap, Minn.)*. 2016;22(1Epilepsy):51–9.

5. IE Scheffer and SF Berkovic. Generalized epilepsy with febrile seizures plus: A genetic disorder with heterogeneous clinical phenotypes. *Brain*. 1997;120 (pt. 3):479–90.

6. YH Zhang, R Burgess, JP Malone et al. Genetic epilepsy with febrile seizures plus: Refining the spectrum. *Neurology*. 2017;89(12):1210–19.

7. LG Epstein, S Shinnar, DC Hesdorffer et al. Human herpesvirus 6 and 7 in febrile status epilepticus: The FEBSTAT study. *Epilepsia*. 2012;53(9):1481–8.

8. DV Lewis, S Shinnar, DC Hesdorffer et al. Hippocampal sclerosis after febrile status epilepticus: The FEBSTAT study. *Ann Neurol*. 2014;75(2):178–85.

9. KB Nelson and JH Ellenberg. Predictors of epilepsy in children who have experienced febrile seizures. *N Engl J Med*. 1976;295(19):1029–33.

10. Subcommittee on Febrile Seizures, American Academy of Pediatrics. Neurodiagnostic evaluation of the child with a simple febrile seizure. *Pediatrics*. 2011;127(2):389–94.

11. DR Nordli, Jr., SL Moshe, S Shinnar et al. Acute EEG findings in children with febrile status epilepticus: Results of the FEBSTAT study. *Neurology*. 2012;79(22):2180–6.

12. DC Hesdorffer, EK Benn, E Bagiella et al. Distribution of febrile seizure duration and associations with development. *Ann Neurol*. 2011;70(1):93–100.

13. E Pavlidou and C Panteliadis. Prognostic factors for subsequent epilepsy in children with febrile seizures. *Epilepsia*. 2013;54(12):2101–7.

14. N Specchio, E Wirrell, IE Scheffer et al. International League Against Epilepsy classification and definition of epilepsy syndromes with onset in childhood: Position paper by the ILAE Task Force on Nosology and Definitions. *Epilepsia*. 2022; 63(6):1398–442.

15. SM Zuberi, E Wirrell, E Yosawitz et al. ILAE classification and definition of epilepsy syndromes in the neonates and infants: Position statement by the ILAE Task Force on Nosology and Definitions. *Epilepsia*. 2022; 63(6):1349–97.

16. JD Symonds, KS Elliott, J Shetty et al. Early childhood epilepsies: Epidemiology, classification, aetiology, genomics, socio-economic determinants. *Brain*. 2021;144(9):2879–91.

17. O Devinsky, JH Cross, and S Wright. Trial of cannabidiol for drug-resistant seizures in the Dravet syndrome. *N Engl J Med*. 2017;377(7):699–700.

18. C Chiron, MC Marchand, A Tran et al. Stiripentol in severe myoclonic epilepsy in infancy: A randomised placebo-controlled syndrome-dedicated trial. STICLO Study Group. *Lancet*. 2000;356(9242):1638–42.

19. R Nabbout, A Mistry, S Zuberi et al. Fenfluramine for treatment-resistant seizures in patients with Dravet syndrome receiving stiripentol-inclusive regimens: A randomized clinical trial. *JAMA Neurol*. 2020;77(3):300–8.

20. J Klepper, C Akman, M Armeno et al. Glut1 deficiency syndrome (Glut1DS): State of the art in 2020 and recommendations of the International Glut1DS Study Group. *Epilepsia Open*. 2020;5(3):354–65.

21. O Devinsky, AD Patel, JH Cross et al. Effect of cannabidiol on drop seizures in the Lennox–Gastaut syndrome. *N Engl J Med*. 2018;378(20):1888–97.

22. S Koh, E Wirrell, A Vezzani et al. Proposal to optimize evaluation and treatment of Febrile infection-related epilepsy syndrome (FIRES): A report from FIRES workshop. *Epilepsia Open*. 2021;6(1):62–72.

23. CP Panayiotopoulos, M Michael, S Sanders, T Valeta, and M Koutroumanidis. Benign childhood focal epilepsies: Assessment of established and newly recognized syndromes. *Brain*. 2008;131(pt. 9):2264–86.

24. IE Scheffer, S Berkovic, G Capovilla et al. ILAE classification of the epilepsies: Position paper of the ILAE Commission for Classification and Terminology. *Epilepsia*. 2017;58(4):512–21.

25. E Wyllie, BE Gidal, HP Goodkin, L Jehi, and T Loddenkemper. *Wyllie's Treatment of Epilepsy: Principles and Practice*. Philadelphia: Wolters Kluwer; 2020.

26. E Hirsch, J French, IE Scheffer et al. ILAE definition of the idiopathic generalized epilepsy syndromes: Position statement by the ILAE Task Force on Nosology and Definitions. *Epilepsia*. 2022;63(6):1475–99.

27. DA Krueger, H Northrup, and International Tuberous Sclerosis Complex Consensus Group. Tuberous sclerosis complex surveillance and management: Recommendations of the 2012 International Tuberous Sclerosis Complex Consensus Conference. *Pediatr Neurol*. 2013;49(4):255–65.

28. S Sabeti, KL Ball, SK Bhattacharya et al. Consensus statement for the management and treatment of Sturge–Weber syndrome: Neurology, neuroimaging, and ophthalmology recommendations. *Pediatr Neurol*. 2021;121:59–66.

29. N Salamon, M Andres, DJ Chute et al. Contralateral hemimicrencephaly and clinical-pathological correlations in children with hemimegalencephaly. *Brain*. 2006;129(pt. 2):352–65.

30. AJ Barkovich, R Guerrini, RI Kuzniecky, GD Jackson, and WB Dobyns. A developmental and genetic classification for malformations of cortical development: Update 2012. *Brain*. 2012;135(pt. 5):1348–69.

31. AM Devlin, JH Cross, W Harkness et al. Clinical outcomes of hemispherectomy for epilepsy in childhood and adolescence. *Brain*. 2003;126(pt. 3):556–66.

32. CG Bien, T Granata, C Antozzi et al. Pathogenesis, diagnosis and treatment of Rasmussen encephalitis: A European consensus statement. *Brain*. 2005;128(pt. 3):454–71.

33. CG Bien, H Tiemeier, R Sassen et al. Rasmussen encephalitis: Incidence and course under randomized therapy with tacrolimus or intravenous immunoglobulins. *Epilepsia*. 2013;54(3):543–50.

34. S Varadkar, CG Bien, CA Kruse et al. Rasmussen's encephalitis: Clinical features, pathobiology, and treatment advances. *Lancet Neurol*. 2014;13(2):195–205.

35. YM Hart, F Andermann, Y Robitaille et al. Double pathology in Rasmussen's syndrome: A window on the etiology? *Neurology*. 1998;50(3):731–5.

36. H Takei, A Wilfong, A Malphrus et al. Dual pathology in Rasmussen's encephalitis: A study of seven cases and review of the literature. *Neuropathology*. 2010;30(4):381–91.

37. CG Bien and J Schramm. Treatment of Rasmussen encephalitis half a century after its initial description: Promising prospects and a dilemma. *Epilepsy Res.* 2009;86(2–3):101–12.

Index